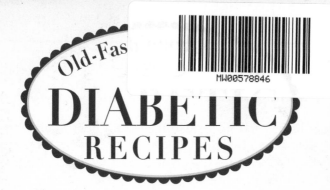

Old-Fas...

DIABETIC
RECIPES

Introduction

Have You Heard the Good News?

You don't have to be a prisoner to diabetes. Once you indulge in these delicious dishes from *Old-Fashioned Favorite Diabetic Recipes,* you'll be amazed that meals so good for you can be so scrumptious. From breakfast treats to light lunches, dinners, desserts and more, this wonderful collection of recipes is sure to be enormously helpful in successfully managing your diabetes.

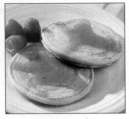
page 6

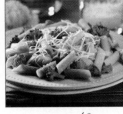
page 40

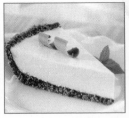
page 76

Nutritional Analyses

Each recipe comes with the nutritional information you need to determine how the food will affect your blood sugar, as well as how it will fit with your calorie, fat and sodium goals. This information can also help you mix and match foods within a meal and throughout your day for optimum health and control over your diabetes. The nutritional values for the recipes in this book were calculated by an independent nutrition consulting firm. The Dietary Exchanges are based on the Exchange Lists for Meal Planning, developed by the American Diabetes Association, Inc. and the American Dietetic Association.

Introduction

Every effort has been made to check the accuracy of these numbers. However, because numerous variables account for a wide range of values in certain foods, all analyses that appear in the book should be considered approximate. Unless otherwise specified, the nutritional calculations were also based on the following:

• Each analysis is based on a single serving of the recipe.

• Optional ingredients and garnishes were not included.

• If a range is given for an ingredient, the lesser amount was used. If an ingredient is presented with an option (e.g., 2 cups hot cooked rice or noodles), the first item listed was the one used.

• In photographs, extra foods shown on the same serving plate with the food of interest were not included.

• Meats were trimmed of all visible fat. Cooked rice, pasta and noodles were prepared without added salt and fat.

• Because Carbohydrate Counting is the method being taught by so many registered dietitians and certified diabetes educators today, sugar amounts are not listed in the nutritional analyses. Instead, total carbohydrate amounts are given. Some of the recipe titles in this publication are marked with a helpful carbohydrate-friendly icon. It appears with any recipe containing 30 grams or less of carbohydrate per serving.

• Goals for healthful eating are based on total foods consumed throughout the day and over a period of time—not just on particular foods. Because of this, a range of healthful recipes with varying nutritional values are included within this book.

• Moderation, portion sizes and meal planning are the keys to success with any healthful eating plan.

Breakfast

Ham and Vegetable Omelet

    Nonstick cooking spray
2 ounces diced 95% fat-free ham (about ½ cup)
1 small onion, diced
½ medium green bell pepper, diced
½ medium red bell pepper, diced
2 cloves garlic, minced
1½ cups cholesterol-free egg substitute
⅛ teaspoon black pepper
½ cup (2 ounces) shredded reduced-fat Colby
    cheese, divided
1 medium tomato, chopped
    Hot pepper sauce (optional)

1. Spray 12-inch nonstick skillet with cooking spray; heat over medium-high heat. Add ham, onion, bell peppers and garlic; cook and stir 5 minutes or until vegetables are crisp-tender. Transfer mixture to large bowl; set aside.

2. Wipe out skillet with paper towels; spray again with cooking spray. Heat over medium-high heat. Pour egg substitute into skillet; sprinkle with black pepper. Cook over medium-high heat about 2 minutes or until bottom is set, lifting edge of egg with spatula to allow uncooked portion to flow underneath. Reduce heat to medium-low. Cover; cook 4 minutes or until top of egg is set.

3. Gently slide omelet onto large serving plate; spoon reserved ham mixture down center of omelet. Sprinkle with ¼ cup cheese. Carefully fold 2 opposite sides of omelet over ham mixture to cover. Sprinkle with

remaining ¼ cup cheese and tomato. Cut into 4 wedges;
serve immediately with hot pepper sauce, if desired.

Makes 4 servings

Nutrients per serving: (1 omelet wedge)

Calories	126	**Carbohydrate**	8 g
Calories from Fat	26 %	**Cholesterol**	17 mg
Total Fat	4 g	**Sodium**	443 mg
Saturated Fat	2 g	**Dietary Fiber**	1 g
Protein	16 g		

Dietary Exchanges: 1 Vegetable, 2 Lean Meat, 1 Fat

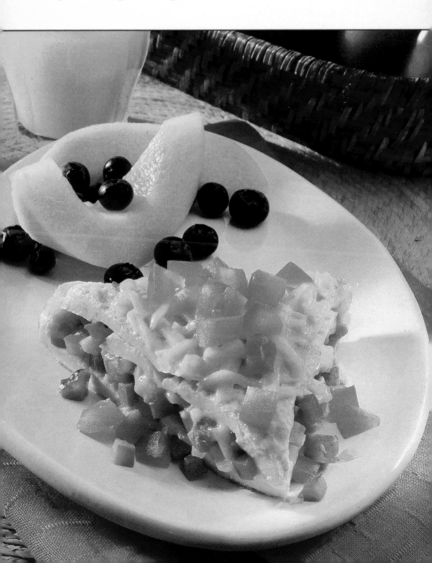

Pumpkin Pancakes

1 cup all-purpose flour
3 tablespoons sugar substitute*
1 teaspoon baking powder
½ teaspoon pumpkin pie spice
¼ teaspoon baking soda
¼ teaspoon salt
¾ cup low-fat buttermilk
½ cup canned solid-pack pumpkin
1 egg
1 tablespoon canola oil
½ teaspoon vanilla
8 tablespoons sugar-free pancake syrup

*This recipe was tested with sucralose-based sugar substitute.

1. Combine flour, sugar substitute, baking powder, pumpkin pie spice, baking soda and salt in medium bowl; mix well. Set aside.

2. Whisk together buttermilk, pumpkin, egg, oil and vanilla in small bowl. Add buttermilk mixture to flour mixture; stir until moist batter forms.

3. Spray griddle or large nonstick skillet with nonstick cooking spray; heat over medium-high heat. Spoon 2 tablespoons batter onto griddle for each pancake; spread batter to 3-inch diameter. Cook 2 to 3 minutes or until bubbles form on surface. Turn and cook about 1 minute more or until bottom is lightly browned. Serve with syrup.   *Makes 8 servings or 16 pancakes*

Pumpkin-Cranberry Pancakes: Add ½ cup fresh or frozen (unthawed) cranberries to batter.

Breakfast

<u>Nutrients per serving:</u> (2 pancakes with 1 tablespoon syrup)

Calories	108	Carbohydrate	18 g
Calories from Fat	23 %	Cholesterol	27 mg
Total Fat	3 g	Sodium	221 mg
Saturated Fat	<1 g	Dietary Fiber	1 g
Protein	3 g		

Dietary Exchanges: 1 Starch, ½ Fat

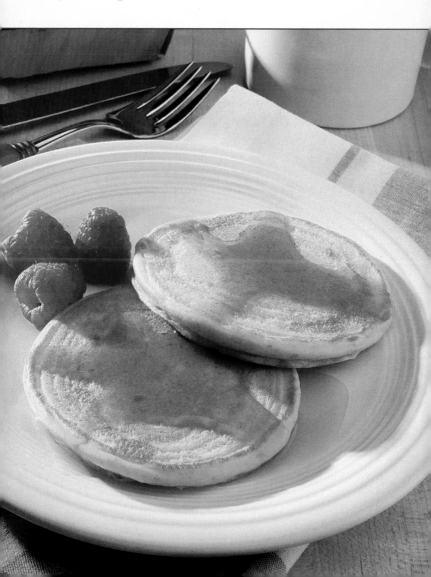

French Toast with Warm Apples

4 egg whites
2 eggs, whole
3 tablespoons sugar substitute,* divided
3 tablespoons fat-free (skim) milk
½ teaspoon vanilla, divided
⅛ teaspoon ground nutmeg
5 ounces Italian bread, cut diagonally into
    4 slices
  Nonstick cooking spray
2 teaspoons canola oil
1 cup sliced unpeeled Granny Smith apples
2 tablespoons water
1 tablespoon reduced-fat margarine
4 teaspoons sugar-free pancake syrup

This recipe was tested with sucralose-based sugar substitute.

1. Combine egg whites, eggs, 2 tablespoons sugar substitute, milk, ¼ teaspoon vanilla and nutmeg in 13×9-inch baking dish; stir with fork until well blended. Add bread slices; turn several times to coat evenly.

2. Coat medium nonstick skillet with cooking spray. Add oil; heat over medium heat. Tilt skillet to coat with oil. Add bread slices; cook 3 minutes. Turn; cook 3 minutes longer or until golden. Remove from skillet; keep warm.

3. Meanwhile, combine apples, water and remaining 1 tablespoon sugar substitute in small skillet; bring to a boil over medium heat. Reduce heat; simmer, uncovered, 2 minutes or until apples are just crisp-tender. Remove from heat; add margarine and remaining ¼ teaspoon vanilla, stirring until margarine is melted.

Breakfast

4. Top each bread slice with 1 teaspoon syrup and equal amounts of apple mixture. *Makes 4 (1-slice) servings*

Nutrients per serving: (1 slice French toast with ¼ cup apple mixture)

Calories	221	Carbohydrate	31 g
Calories from Fat	34 %	Cholesterol	106 mg
Total Fat	8 g	Sodium	349 mg
Saturated Fat	2 g	Dietary Fiber	1 g
Protein	11 g		

Dietary Exchanges: 2 Starch, 1½ Lean Meat, 1½ Fat

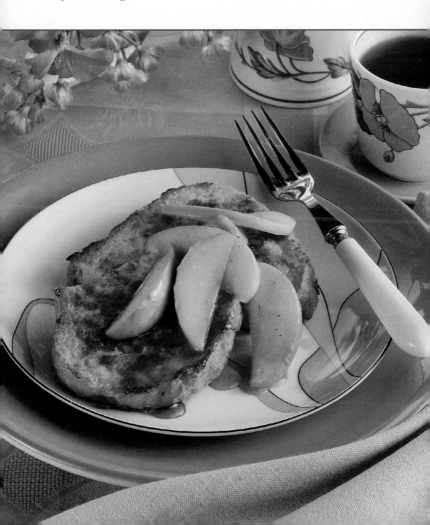

Peach Pecan Upside-Down Cake

2 tablespoons butter, melted
2 tablespoons packed light brown sugar
1 tablespoon maple syrup
8 ounces frozen unsweetened peach slices, thawed
3 tablespoons pecan pieces
⅔ cup biscuit baking mix
2 eggs
⅓ cup fat-free (skim) milk
½ teaspoon vanilla

1. Preheat oven to 400°F. Spray 8- or 9-inch pie pan with nonstick cooking spray.

2. Pour butter into prepared pan. Sprinkle with brown sugar and maple syrup. Arrange peach slices in single layer on top in decorative circle. Sprinkle with pecans.

3. Place baking mix in medium bowl. Whisk together eggs, milk and vanilla in small bowl; stir into baking mix just until moistened. Pour batter over peaches.

4. Bake 15 to 18 minutes or until lightly browned and toothpick inserted into center comes out clean. Cool 1 minute. Run knife around outer edge of pan. Invert cake onto serving plate. Cut into 6 wedges.

Makes 6 servings

Breakfast

<u>Nutrients per serving:</u> (1 cake wedge [⅙ of total recipe])

Calories	175	Carbohydrate	20 g
Calories from Fat	47 %	Cholesterol	82 mg
Total Fat	9 g	Sodium	223 mg
Saturated Fat	4 g	Dietary Fiber	<1 g
Protein	4 g		

Dietary Exchanges: 1 Starch, ½ Fruit, 1½ Fat

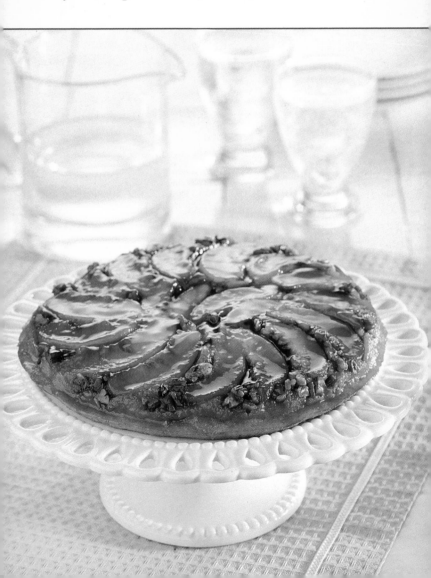

Breakfast Sandwiches

Carb Friendly

**4 turkey breakfast sausage patties (about
    4 ounces total)**
1½ cups cholesterol-free egg substitute
½ cup fat-free (skim) milk
2 tablespoons sliced green onion
¼ teaspoon black pepper
⅛ teaspoon salt (optional)
4 English muffins, split and toasted
**2 tablespoons shredded reduced-fat sharp
    Cheddar cheese**

1. Heat large skillet over medium-high heat. Crumble sausage patties into skillet. Brown sausage, stirring to break up meat; drain fat.

2. Whisk egg substitute, milk, green onion, pepper and salt, if desired, in medium bowl. Pour over sausage in skillet. Cook, without stirring, over medium heat until mixture begins to set. Using spatula, lift egg mixture, allowing uncooked portion to flow underneath. Continue cooking until egg mixture is set but still moist.

3. Immediately spoon egg mixture onto toasted English muffin halves. Sprinkle with cheese. Cover loosely with foil. Let stand about 30 seconds or until cheese melts.

Makes 4 servings

Nutrients per serving: (2 open-faced sandwiches [2 English muffin halves with ¾ cup egg mixture])

Calories	288	Carbohydrate	28 g
Calories from Fat	30 %	Cholesterol	25 mg
Total Fat	9 g	Sodium	575 mg
Saturated Fat	1 g	Dietary Fiber	1 g
Protein	23 g		

Dietary Exchanges: 2 Starch, 3 Lean Meat, 2 Fat

Cherry-Orange Oatmeal

1 can (11 ounces) mandarin orange segments
   in light syrup, rinsed and drained
1 cup fresh pitted cherries or frozen dark sweet
   cherries
2 cups water
1 cup uncooked old-fashioned oats
2 tablespoons sugar substitute*
1 tablespoon unsweetened cocoa powder

*This recipe was tested with sucralose-based sugar
substitute.*

MICROWAVE DIRECTIONS
1. Set aside 8 orange segments and 4 cherries for
garnish. Combine water, remaining orange segments,
cherries, oats, sugar substitute and cocoa in 1½-quart
microwavable casserole. Microwave on HIGH 2 minutes.
Stir; microwave 4 minutes.

2. Divide evenly among 4 serving bowls. Garnish with
reserved oranges and cherries.   *Makes 4 servings*

Nutrients per serving: (¾ cup oatmeal with garnish of
2 orange segments and 1 cherry)

Calories	150	Carbohydrate	39 g
Calories from Fat	11 %	Cholesterol	0 mg
Total Fat	2 g	Sodium	6 mg
Saturated Fat	<1 g	Dietary Fiber	3 g
Protein	4 g		

Dietary Exchanges: 1 Starch, 1½ Fruit

Lunch

Tuna Melts

1 can (12 ounces) reduced-sodium chunk white tuna packed in water, drained and flaked
1½ cups coleslaw mix
3 tablespoons sliced green onions
3 tablespoons reduced-fat mayonnaise
1 tablespoon Dijon mustard
1 teaspoon dried dill weed (optional)
4 English muffins, split and lightly toasted
⅓ cup shredded reduced-fat Cheddar cheese

1. Preheat broiler. Combine tuna, coleslaw mix and green onions in medium bowl. Combine mayonnaise, mustard and dill weed, if desired, in small bowl. Stir mayonnaise mixture into tuna mixture. Spread tuna mixture onto muffin halves. Place on broiler pan.

2. Broil 4 inches from heat 3 to 4 minutes or until heated through. Sprinkle with cheese. Broil 1 to 2 minutes more or until cheese is melted.   *Makes 4 servings*

Nutrients per serving: (2 melts [2 topped muffin halves])

Calories	294	**Carbohydrate**	29 g
Calories from Fat	19 %	**Cholesterol**	31 mg
Total Fat	6 g	**Sodium**	459 mg
Saturated Fat	1 g	**Dietary Fiber**	2 g
Protein	29 g		

Dietary Exchanges: 2 Starch, 4 Lean Meat, 1 Fat

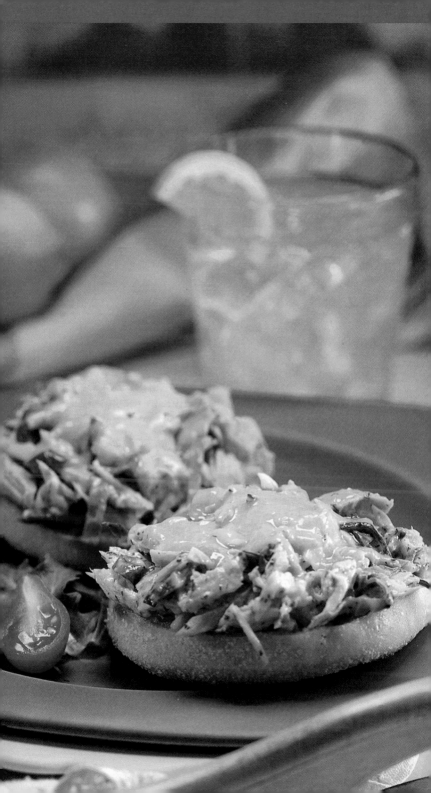

Mexican Pita Pile-Ups

4 (4-inch) rounds whole wheat pita bread
1 cup shredded cooked boneless skinless
    chicken breast
¼ cup canned chopped mild green chiles,
    drained
1 tablespoon fresh lime juice
1 teaspoon ground cumin
1 cup chopped seeded fresh tomato
¼ cup chopped fresh cilantro (optional)
1 can (2¼ ounces) sliced ripe olives, drained
1 cup (4 ounces) shredded reduced-fat sharp
    Cheddar cheese

MICROWAVE DIRECTIONS

1. Place pita rounds on microwavable plates. Combine chicken, chiles, lime juice and cumin in medium bowl. Top pitas evenly with chicken mixture, tomato, cilantro, if desired, olives and cheese.

2. Microwave each pile-up on HIGH 1 minute or until cheese is melted. Let stand 2 to 3 minutes or until crust is slightly firm. *Makes 4 servings*

Nutrients per serving: (1 pile-up)

Calories	258	Carbohydrate	20 g
Calories from Fat	36%	Cholesterol	50 mg
Total Fat	10 g	Sodium	579 mg
Saturated Fat	5 g	Dietary Fiber	3 g
Protein	21 g		

Dietary Exchanges: 1½ Starch, 3½ Lean Meat, 2 Fat

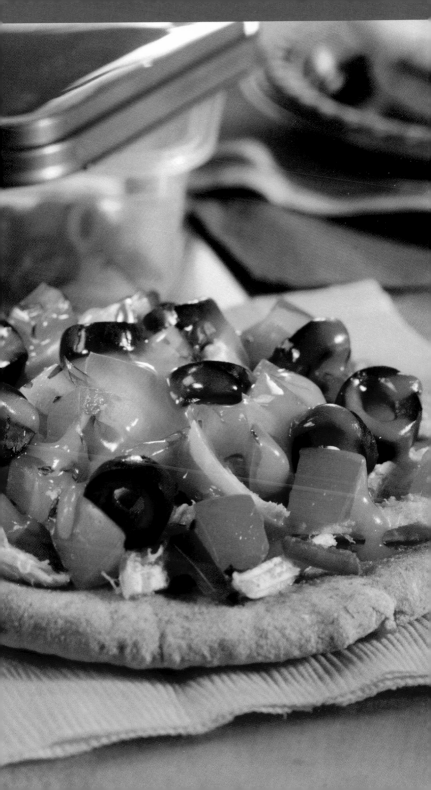

Chunky Chicken and Vegetable Soup

1 tablespoon canola oil

1 boneless skinless chicken breast (about ¼ pound), diced

½ cup chopped green bell pepper

½ cup thinly sliced celery

2 green onions, sliced

2 cans (about 14 ounces each) fat-free reduced-sodium chicken broth

1 cup water

½ cup sliced carrots

2 tablespoons reduced-fat whipping cream

⅛ teaspoon black pepper

1 tablespoon finely chopped fresh parsley (optional)

¼ teaspoon dried thyme (optional)

1. Heat oil in large saucepan over medium heat. Add chicken; cook and stir 4 to 5 minutes or until cooked through. Add bell pepper, celery and onions. Cook and stir 7 minutes or until vegetables are tender.

2. Add broth, water, carrots, cream, black pepper and parsley and thyme, if desired. Simmer 10 minutes or until carrots are tender. *Makes 4 servings*

Nutrients per serving: (1 bowl of soup [¼ of total recipe])

Calories	104	Carbohydrate	4 g
Calories from Fat	52%	Cholesterol	25 mg
Total Fat	6 g	Sodium	480 mg
Saturated Fat	2 g	Dietary Fiber	1 g
Protein	8 g		

Dietary Exchanges: 1 Vegetable, 1 Lean Meat, 1½ Fat

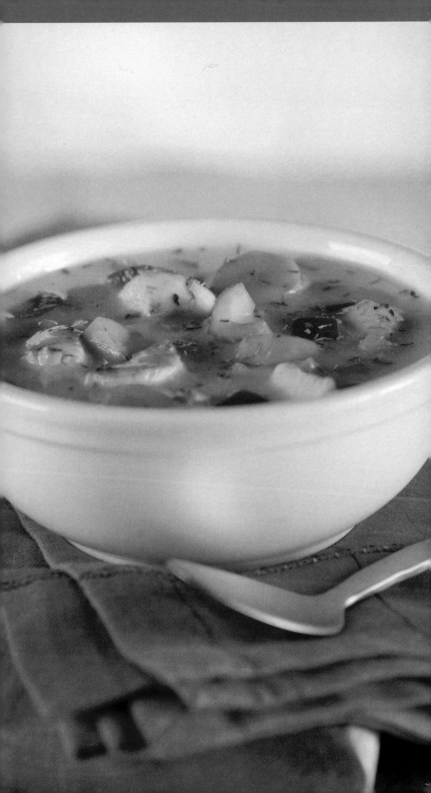

Grilled Salmon Salad

⅓ cup plus 2 tablespoons fat-free raspberry or balsamic vinaigrette salad dressing, divided

4 skinless salmon fillets (about ¼ pound each and ¾ inch thick)

½ teaspoon black pepper

¼ teaspoon salt

8 cups spring mix salad greens

2 cups cherry tomatoes, cut into halves

¼ cup fresh basil leaves, chopped or julienned (optional)

1. Prepare grill for direct cooking. Brush 2 tablespoons dressing over salmon fillets. Sprinkle with pepper and salt. Grill, covered, over medium-high heat 5 to 6 minutes or until salmon begins to flake when tested with fork. (Do not overcook or salmon will become dry.)

2. Meanwhile, combine greens, tomatoes and remaining ⅓ cup dressing in large bowl. Transfer to plates. Top with salmon; sprinkle with basil, if desired.

Makes 4 servings

Note: To broil the salmon, preheat broiler. Place salmon on an oiled broiler pan. Broil 4 inches from heat 6 to 7 minutes or just until the salmon begins to flake when tested with fork.

<u>**Nutrients per serving:**</u> (1 salmon fillet with ¼ of salad mixture)

Calories	264	Carbohydrate	12 g
Calories from Fat	44%	Cholesterol	66 mg
Total Fat	12 g	Sodium	493 mg
Saturated Fat	2 g	Dietary Fiber	3 g
Protein	24 g		

Dietary Exchanges: 2 Vegetable, 3 Lean Meat, 2 Fat

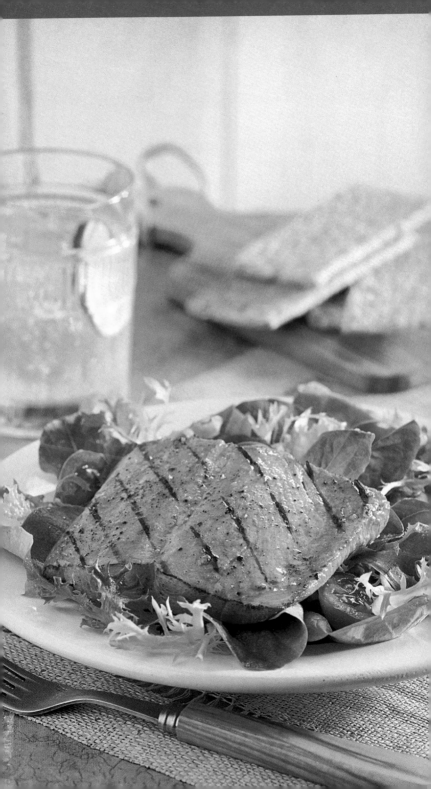

Diner Egg Salad Sandwiches

6 eggs
2 tablespoons fat-free mayonnaise
1 tablespoon plus 1½ teaspoons sweet pickle relish
½ cup finely chopped celery
⅛ to ¼ teaspoon salt
Black pepper (optional)
8 slices whole-grain bread

1. Place eggs in medium saucepan. Add enough cold water to cover eggs. Bring to a boil over high heat. Immediately reduce heat; simmer 10 minutes. Drain and peel eggs under cold water.

2. Cut eggs in half. Discard 4 yolk halves or reserve for another use. Place remaining egg yolks in medium bowl. Add mayonnaise and pickle relish. Mash with fork until yolk mixture is well blended and creamy. Chop egg whites; add to yolk mixture with celery and salt. Stir until well blended. Season with pepper, if desired.

3. Spread ½ cup egg salad on each of 4 bread slices; top with remaining bread. Slice sandwiches in half, if desired, before serving. *Makes 4 servings*

Nutrients per serving: (1 sandwich [2 halves])

Calories	253	Carbohydrate	28 g
Calories from Fat	34 %	Cholesterol	318 mg
Total Fat	10 g	Sodium	551 mg
Saturated Fat	3 g	Dietary Fiber	4 g
Protein	15 g		

Dietary Exchanges: 2 Starch, 2 Lean Meat, 2 Fat

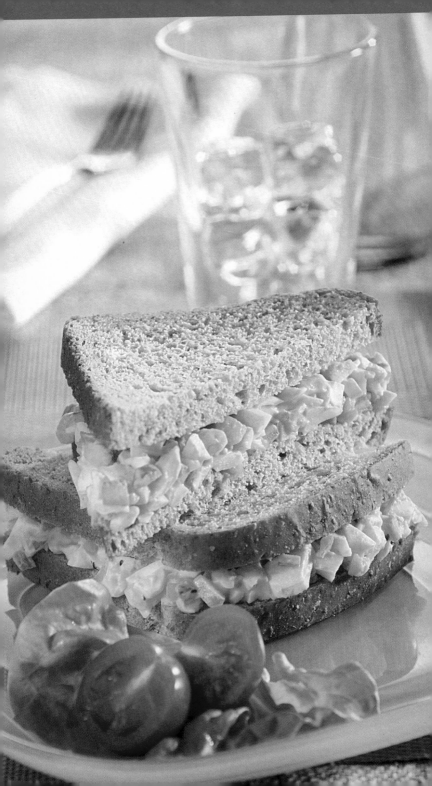

Grilled Salsa Turkey Burger

3 ounces 93% lean ground turkey
1 tablespoon mild or medium salsa
1 tablespoon crushed baked tortilla chips
1 slice (1 ounce) reduced-fat Monterey Jack
    cheese (optional)
1 whole wheat hamburger bun, split
    Green leaf lettuce
    Additional salsa (optional)

1. Lightly spray grid with nonstick cooking spray to prevent sticking. Prepare grill for direct cooking. Combine turkey, 1 tablespoon salsa and chips in small bowl; mix lightly. Shape into patty.

2. Grill burger over medium-high heat 6 minutes per side or until cooked through (165°F). Top with cheese, if desired, during last 2 minutes of grilling time. Place bun, cut sides down, on grill during last 2 minutes of grilling to lightly brown.

3. Cover bottom half of bun with lettuce; top with burger, additional salsa, if desired, and top half of bun.

Makes 1 serving

Note: To broil, preheat broiler. Broil burger 4 to 6 inches from heat 6 minutes per side or until cooked through (165°F).

Nutrients per serving: (1 sandwich [without cheese])

Calories	302	Carbohydrate	29 g
Calories from Fat	33%	Cholesterol	63 mg
Total Fat	11 g	Sodium	494 mg
Saturated Fat	3 g	Dietary Fiber	2 g
Protein	22 g		

Dietary Exchanges: 2 Starch, 3 Lean Meat, 2 Fat

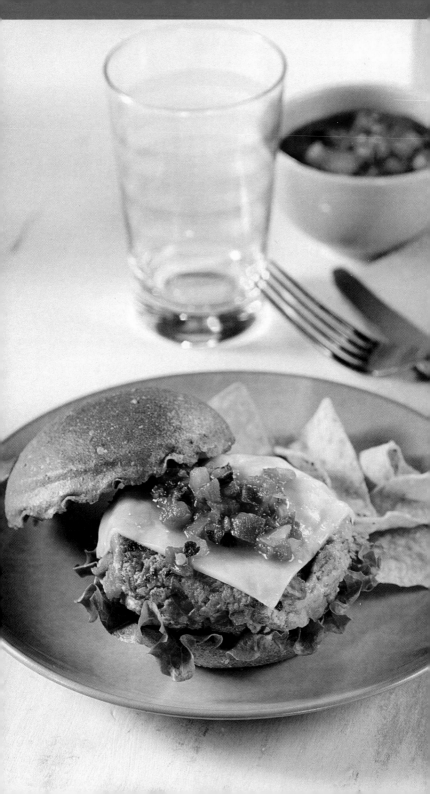

Mediterranean Tuna Sandwiches

1 can (12 ounces) reduced-sodium solid white tuna packed in water, drained
¼ cup finely chopped red onion
¼ cup fat-free or reduced-fat mayonnaise
3 tablespoons chopped ripe olives, drained
1 tablespoon plus 1 teaspoon lemon juice
1 tablespoon chopped fresh mint (optional)
1 tablespoon olive oil
¼ teaspoon black pepper
⅛ teaspoon garlic powder (optional)
4 thin slices tomato
8 slices whole wheat bread

1. Combine tuna, onion, mayonnaise, olives, lemon juice, mint, if desired, olive oil, pepper and garlic powder, if desired, in large bowl until blended.

2. Top each of 4 bread slices with tomato slice. Spoon ⅔ cup tuna mixture over each tomato slice. Top with remaining bread slices. Cut sandwiches in half to serve.

Makes 4 servings

Nutrients per serving: (1 sandwich [2 halves])

Calories	332	Carbohydrate	27 g
Calories from Fat	33 %	Cholesterol	31 mg
Total Fat	12 g	Sodium	483 mg
Saturated Fat	2 g	Dietary Fiber	4 g
Protein	29 g		

Dietary Exchanges: 1½ Starch, ½ Vegetable, 4 Lean Meat, 2 Fat

Crunch Cobb Salad with Blue Cheese and Peas

6 cups torn mixed salad greens
1 cup frozen green peas, thawed
1 cup cucumber slices
1 cup chopped or sliced bell pepper
¼ cup chopped or sliced red onion
½ cup fat-free vinaigrette
3 ounces smoked turkey, diced or thinly sliced
2 ounces extra-lean baked deli ham, diced or thinly sliced
1½ ounces crumbled blue cheese

1. Combine salad greens, peas, cucumber, bell pepper, onion and vinaigrette in large bowl; toss gently to coat.

2. Add turkey, ham and cheese; toss gently.

Makes 4 servings

Tip: To thaw peas quickly, place in a colander and run under cold water 25 seconds. Shake off excess water.

Note: Check labels on turkey and ham for sodium content. Not all sodium levels for lean meats are the same. Brands vary, so look for the product with the least amount of sodium.

Nutrients per serving: (2 cups salad)

Calories	170	Carbohydrate	19 g
Calories from Fat	26%	Cholesterol	30 mg
Total Fat	5 g	Sodium	608 mg
Saturated Fat	2 g	Dietary Fiber	4 g
Protein	14 g		

Dietary Exchanges: ½ Starch, 2½ Vegetable, 1½ Lean Meat, 1 Fat

Sausage Vegetable Rotini Soup

   Nonstick cooking spray
  6 ounces bulk pork sausage
  1 cup chopped onion
  1 cup chopped green bell pepper
  3 cups water
  1 can (about 14 ounces) no-salt-added
       diced tomatoes
 ¼ cup reduced-sodium ketchup
  2 teaspoons sodium-free beef bouillon granules
  2 teaspoons chili powder (optional)
  4 ounces uncooked tri-colored rotini pasta
  1 cup frozen corn, thawed and drained

1. Spray Dutch oven with cooking spray. Heat over medium-high heat. Add sausage; cook 3 minutes or until no longer pink, stirring to break up sausage. Drain fat. Add onion and bell pepper; cook and stir 3 to 4 minutes or until onion is translucent.

2. Add water, tomatoes, ketchup, beef bouillon and chili powder, if desired; bring to a boil over high heat. Stir in pasta; return to a boil. Reduce heat to medium-low; simmer, uncovered, 12 minutes. Stir in corn; cook 2 minutes.   *Makes 4 servings*

Nutrients per serving: (about 1⅔ cups soup)

Calories	311	Carbohydrate	45 g
Calories from Fat	26%	Cholesterol	31 mg
Total Fat	9 g	Sodium	272 mg
Saturated Fat	2 g	Dietary Fiber	4 g
Protein	14 g		

Dietary Exchanges: 2 Starch, 1½ Vegetable, 2 Lean Meat, 2 Fat

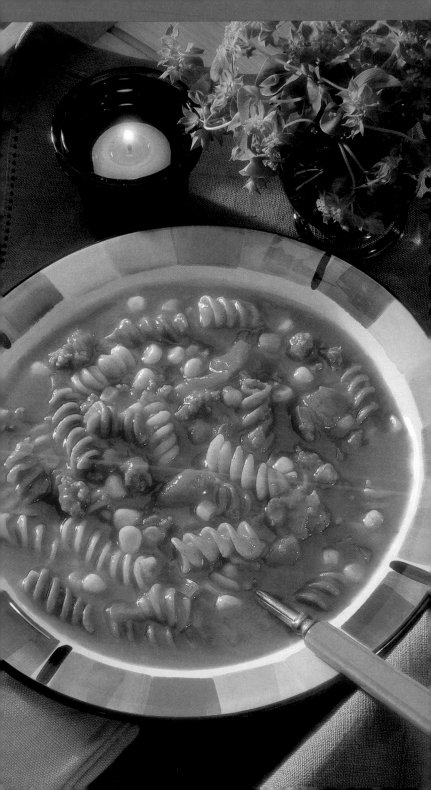

Main-Dish Mediterranean Salad

1 package (10 ounces) ready-to-use chopped
   romaine lettuce
½ pound fresh green beans, cooked and drained
   or 1 can (about 14 ounces) whole green
   beans, drained
1 pouch (5½ ounces) solid white tuna, flaked
8 ounces cherry tomatoes, cut into halves
2 tablespoons olive oil
2 tablespoons cider vinegar or white vinegar
1½ teaspoons Dijon mustard
½ teaspoon black pepper

1. Place lettuce, green beans, tuna and tomatoes in large bowl.

2. To make dressing, whisk oil, vinegar, mustard and pepper in small bowl until blended. Pour dressing over salad; toss well. Serve immediately.   *Makes 4 servings*

<u>**Nutrients per serving:**</u> (3 cups salad with dressing)

Calories	156	Carbohydrate	9 g
Calories from Fat	47 %	Cholesterol	18 mg
Total Fat	8 g	Sodium	218 mg
Saturated Fat	1 g	Dietary Fiber	4 g
Protein	13 g		

Dietary Exchanges: 2 Vegetable, 2 Lean Meat, 1½ Fat

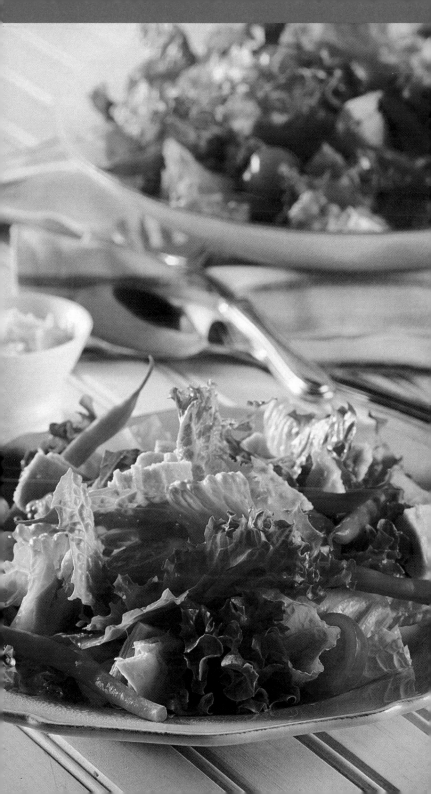

Grilled Mozzarella & Roasted Red Pepper Sandwich

1 tablespoon reduced-fat olive oil vinaigrette or reduced-fat Italian salad dressing

2 slices (1 ounce each) Italian-style sandwich bread

Fresh basil leaves (optional)

⅓ cup roasted red peppers, rinsed, drained and patted dry

2 slices (1 ounce each) part-skim mozzarella or reduced-fat Swiss cheese

Olive oil cooking spray

1. Brush dressing on 1 side of 1 bread slice; top with basil, if desired, peppers, cheese and remaining bread slice. Lightly spray both sides of sandwich with cooking spray.

2. Place large nonstick skillet over medium heat. Add sandwich; cook 4 to 5 minutes per side or until cheese melts and sandwich is golden brown.

Makes 1 sandwich

Nutrients per serving: (1 sandwich)

Calories	303	Carbohydrate	35 g
Calories from Fat	29 %	Cholesterol	25 mg
Total Fat	9 g	Sodium	727 mg
Saturated Fat	5 g	Dietary Fiber	2 g
Protein	16 g		

Dietary Exchanges: 2 Starch, 1 Vegetable, 1 Lean Meat, 1½ Fat

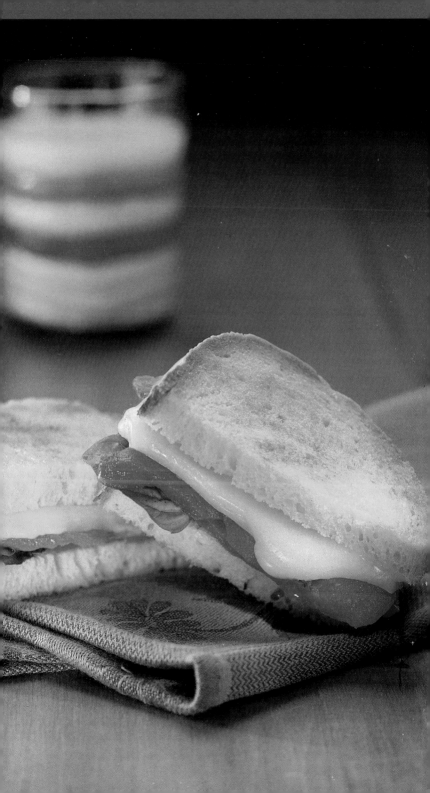

Dinner

Roasted Almond Tilapia

**2 tilapia fillets or Boston scrod fillets
(6 ounces each)**
¼ teaspoon salt
1 tablespoon prepared mustard
¼ cup whole wheat bread crumbs
2 tablespoons chopped unblanched almonds
Paprika (optional)
Lemon wedges (optional)

1. Preheat oven to 450°F. Place fish on small baking sheet; season with salt. Spread mustard over fish. Combine bread crumbs and almonds in small bowl; sprinkle over fish. Press lightly to adhere. Sprinkle with paprika, if desired.

2. Bake 8 to 10 minutes or until fish is opaque in center and just begins to flake when tested with fork. Serve with lemon wedges, if desired.   *Makes 2 servings*

Nutrients per serving: (1 fillet)

Calories	268	**Carbohydrate**	14 g
Calories from Fat	32 %	**Cholesterol**	0 mg
Total Fat	10 g	**Sodium**	587 mg
Saturated Fat	<1 g	**Dietary Fiber**	2 g
Protein	32 g		

Dietary Exchanges: 1 Starch, 4 Lean Meat, 2 Fat

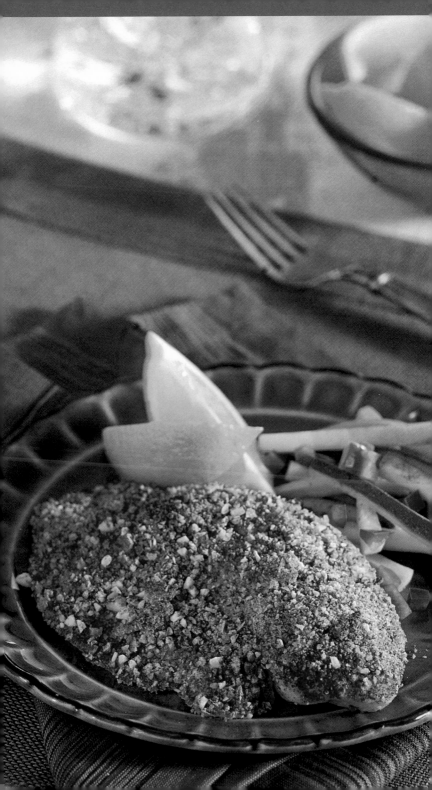

Chicken Roll-Ups

2½ cups reduced-sodium marinara sauce, divided
4 boneless skinless chicken breasts (about ¼ pound each)
2 cups fresh baby spinach leaves
4 slices (1 ounce each) low-moisture part-skim mozzarella cheese
¼ cup grated Parmesan cheese
Red pepper flakes (optional)

1. Preheat oven to 400°F. Spray 2-quart baking dish with nonstick cooking spray. Spread 1 cup marinara sauce on bottom of baking dish.

2. Place 1 chicken breast between 2 sheets of plastic wrap on cutting board. Pound with rolling pin until meat is about ¼ inch thick. Repeat with remaining chicken.

3. Place ½ cup spinach leaves on each chicken breast. Top with mozzarella cheese slices. Roll up tightly. Place rolls, seam side down, in baking dish. Cover evenly with remaining 1½ cups marinara sauce.

4. Cover dish with foil; bake 35 minutes. Uncover and bake 10 minutes more. Sprinkle with Parmesan cheese; season with red pepper flakes, if desired.

Makes 4 servings

<u>**Nutrients per serving:**</u> (1 roll-up)

Calories	287	Carbohydrate	11 g
Calories from Fat	36%	Cholesterol	85 mg
Total Fat	10 g	Sodium	414 mg
Saturated Fat	5 g	Dietary Fiber	2 g
Protein	37 g		

Dietary Exchanges: 1 Vegetable, ½ Milk, 5 Lean Meat, 2 Fat

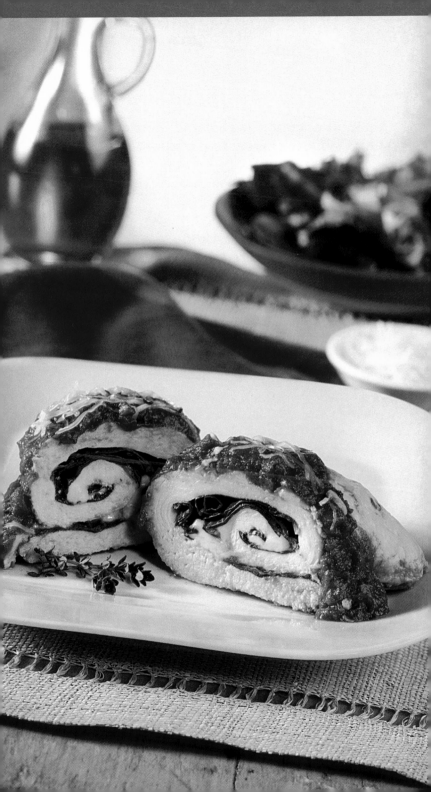

Italian-Style Shepherd's Pie

- **1 pound potatoes, peeled and quartered**
- **2 to 3 tablespoons fat-free reduced-sodium chicken broth**
- **3 tablespoons grated Parmesan cheese**
- **1 pound 95% lean ground beef**
- **½ cup chopped onion**
- **2 teaspoons Italian seasoning**
- **⅛ teaspoon ground red pepper**
- **2 cups sliced yellow summer squash**
- **1 can (about 14 ounces) chunky pasta-style tomatoes, drained**
- **1 cup frozen corn**
- **⅓ cup no-salt-added tomato paste**

1. Preheat oven to 375°F. Combine potatoes and enough water to cover in medium saucepan; bring to a boil. Boil, uncovered, 20 to 25 minutes or until tender. Drain. Mash potatoes, adding enough chicken broth to make desired consistency. Stir in Parmesan cheese. Set aside.

2. Cook and stir ground beef and onion in large skillet over medium-high heat 6 to 8 minutes or until meat is no longer pink. Drain fat. Stir in Italian seasoning and red pepper. Add squash, tomatoes, corn and tomato paste; mix well. Spoon mixture into 2-quart casserole.

3. Pipe or spoon potatoes over top of casserole. Bake, uncovered, 20 to 25 minutes or until meat mixture is bubbly. Let stand 10 minutes before serving.

Makes 6 servings

Dinner

Nutrients per serving: (1¼ cups meat mixture topped with ⅓ cup potatoes)

Calories	245	Carbohydrate	29 g
Calories from Fat	20 %	Cholesterol	47 mg
Total Fat	6 g	Sodium	401 mg
Saturated Fat	2 g	Dietary Fiber	5 g
Protein	21 g		

Dietary Exchanges: 2 Starch, 3 Lean Meat, 1 Fat

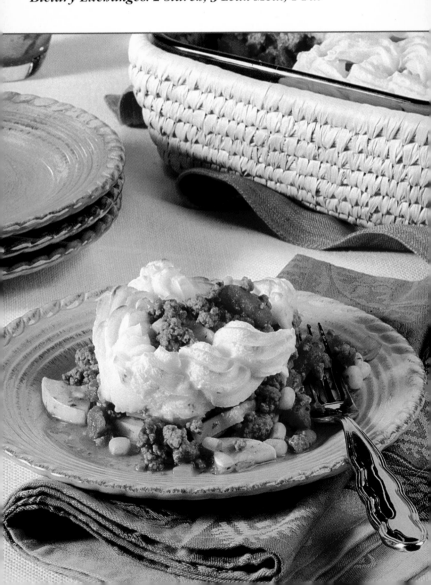

Whole Wheat Penne with Broccoli and Sausage

6 to 7 ounces uncooked whole wheat penne pasta
8 ounces broccoli florets
8 ounces mild Italian turkey sausage, casings removed
1 medium onion, quartered and sliced
2 cloves garlic, minced
2 teaspoons grated lemon peel
¼ teaspoon salt
⅛ teaspoon black pepper
⅓ cup grated Parmesan cheese

1. Cook pasta according to package directions, omitting salt. Add broccoli during last 5 to 6 minutes of cooking. Drain well; cover and keep warm.

2. Meanwhile, heat large nonstick skillet over medium heat. Crumble sausage into skillet. Add onion; cook until sausage is brown, stirring to break up meat. Drain fat.

3. Add garlic; cook and stir 1 minute. Add sausage mixture, lemon peel, salt and pepper to pasta; toss until blended. Sprinkle Parmesan evenly over each serving.

Makes 6 servings

Nutrients per serving: (1⅓ cups)

Calories	208	Carbohydrate	26 g
Calories from Fat	27 %	Cholesterol	26 mg
Total Fat	6 g	Sodium	425 mg
Saturated Fat	1 g	Dietary Fiber	4 g
Protein	13 g		

Dietary Exchanges: 1½ Starch, 1 Vegetable, 2 Lean Meat, 1 Fat

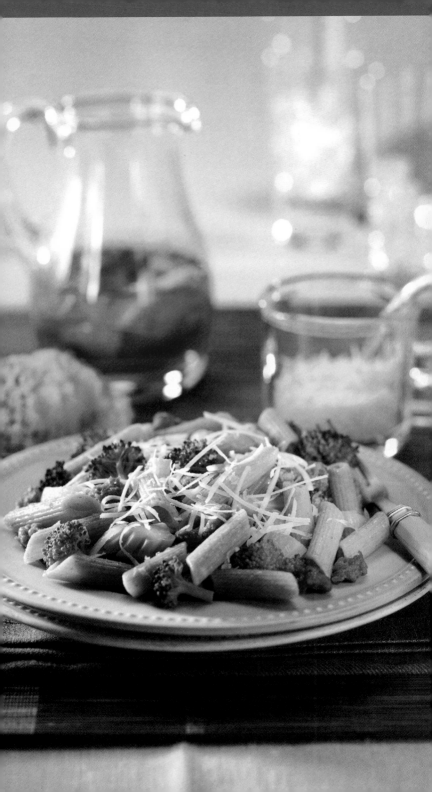

Dinner

Greek Lemon Chicken

4 boneless skinless chicken breasts (about ¼ pound each)
2 tablespoons lemon juice
2 teaspoons extra-virgin olive oil
1 teaspoon grated lemon peel
1 teaspoon dried oregano
1 clove garlic, minced
¼ teaspoon salt
⅛ teaspoon black pepper
   Nonstick cooking spray
1 lemon, cut into wedges (optional)
   Baby spinach leaves (optional)

1. Place chicken in large resealable food storage bag. Add lemon juice, oil, lemon peel, oregano, garlic, salt and pepper. Seal bag. Shake to coat chicken. Refrigerate chicken at least 30 minutes or up to 8 hours.

2. Coat nonstick skillet with cooking spray; heat over medium heat. Add chicken, discarding bag with any remaining marinade. Cook chicken over medium heat 3 minutes. Turn chicken. Reduce heat to medium-low; cook 7 minutes or until no longer pink in center.

3. Remove from heat. Serve with lemon wedges and spinach leaves, if desired. *Makes 4 servings*

Nutrients per serving: (1 breast)

Calories	132	**Carbohydrate**	3 g
Calories from Fat	11%	**Cholesterol**	66 mg
Total Fat	2 g	**Sodium**	74 mg
Saturated Fat	<1 g	**Dietary Fiber**	1 g
Protein	27 g		

Dietary Exchanges: 4 Lean Meat

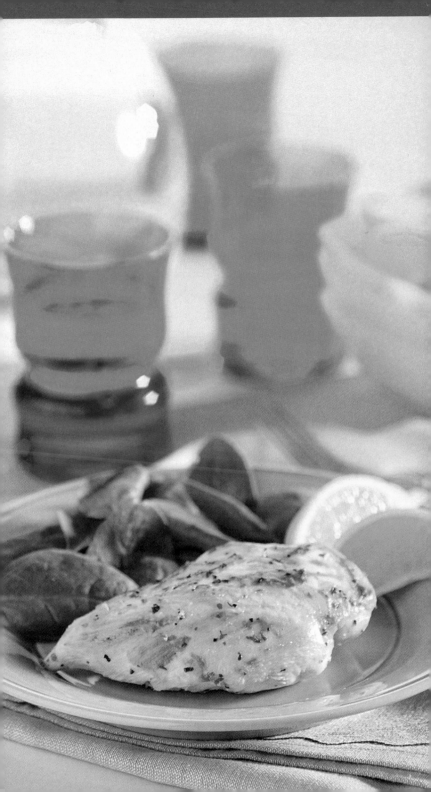

Pork and Sweet Potato Skillet

3/4 **pound pork tenderloin, cut into 1-inch cubes**
1 **tablespoon plus 1 teaspoon butter, divided**
1/4 **teaspoon salt**
1/8 **teaspoon black pepper**
2 **medium sweet potatoes, peeled and cut into**
  1/2-inch pieces (about 2 cups)
1 **small onion, sliced**
1/4 **pound reduced-fat smoked turkey sausage,**
  halved lengthwise and cut into 1/2-inch pieces
1 **small red apple, cored and cut into 1/2-inch**
  pieces
1/2 **cup prepared sweet-and-sour sauce**
2 **tablespoons chopped fresh parsley (optional)**

1. Add pork and 1 teaspoon butter to large nonstick skillet; cook and stir over medium-high heat 2 to 3 minutes or until pork is no longer pink. Season with salt and pepper. Remove from skillet.

2. Add remaining 1 tablespoon butter, potatoes and onion to skillet. Cook and stir over medium-low heat 8 to 10 minutes or until tender.

3. Add pork, turkey sausage, apple and sweet-and-sour sauce to skillet; cook and stir until heated through. Garnish with parsley.   *Makes 4 servings*

Nutrients per serving: (1 1/2 cups)

Calories	309	**Carbohydrate**	39 g
Calories from Fat	22 %	**Cholesterol**	71 mg
Total Fat	7 g	**Sodium**	565 mg
Saturated Fat	4 g	**Dietary Fiber**	3 g
Protein	22 g		

Dietary Exchanges: 2 Starch, 1/2 Fruit, 1/2 Vegetable, 3 Lean Meat, 1 Fat

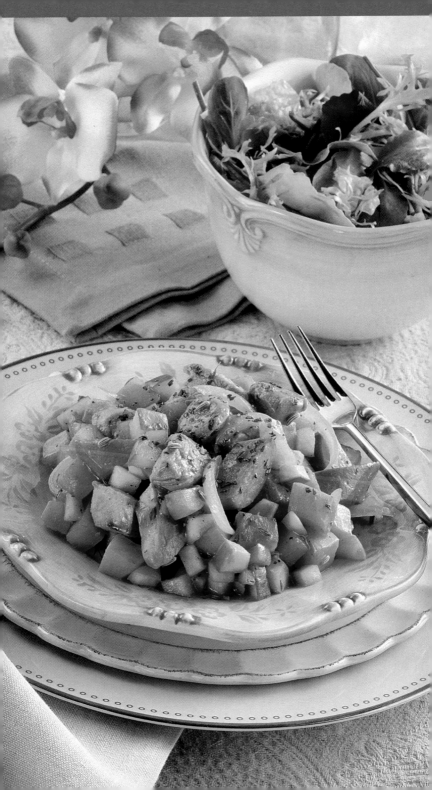

Cajun Chicken Drums

Carb
Friendly

4 chicken drumsticks, skin removed
½ to ¾ teaspoon Cajun seasoning
2 tablespoons lemon juice
½ teaspoon grated lemon peel
½ teaspoon hot pepper sauce
⅛ teaspoon salt
2 tablespoons chopped fresh parsley (optional)

1. Preheat oven to 400°F. Coat shallow baking dish with nonstick cooking spray. Arrange chicken in dish; sprinkle evenly with Cajun seasoning. Cover dish with foil; bake 25 minutes, turning drumsticks once.

2. Remove foil; bake 15 to 20 minutes longer or until cooked through and juices run clear (165°F). Remove from oven. Stir in lemon juice, lemon peel, hot pepper sauce and salt, scraping bottom and sides of baking dish. Sprinkle with parsley, if desired. Serve immediately.

Makes 2 servings

Nutrients per serving: (2 drumsticks)

Calories	173	Carbohydrate	2 g
Calories from Fat	25 %	Cholesterol	108 mg
Total Fat	5 g	Sodium	254 mg
Saturated Fat	1 g	Dietary Fiber	<1 g
Protein	29 g		

Dietary Exchanges: 4 Lean Meat, 1 Fat

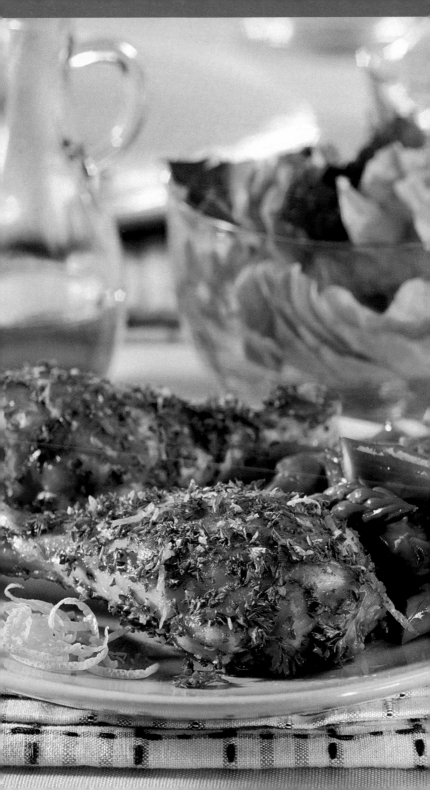

Pork and Plum Kabobs

¾ **pound boneless pork loin chops (1 inch thick), trimmed and cut into 1-inch pieces**
1½ **teaspoons ground cumin**
½ **teaspoon ground cinnamon**
¼ **teaspoon salt**
¼ **teaspoon garlic powder**
¼ **teaspoon ground red pepper**
¼ **cup sliced green onions**
¼ **cup raspberry fruit spread**
1 **tablespoon orange juice**
3 **plums or nectarines, pitted and cut into wedges**
8 **wooden skewers***

Soak wooden skewers in warm water for 30 minutes before using to prevent them from burning.

1. Place pork in large resealable food storage bag. Combine cumin, cinnamon, salt, garlic powder and red pepper in small bowl; add to bag with meat. Seal bag; shake to coat meat with spices.

2. Prepare grill for direct cooking. Combine green onions, raspberry fruit spread and orange juice in small bowl.

3. Alternately thread pork and plum wedges onto 8 skewers. Grill kabobs over medium heat 12 to 14 minutes or until meat is cooked through, turning once. Brush frequently with raspberry mixture during last 5 minutes of grilling.   *Makes 4 servings*

Serving Suggestion: A crisp, cool salad makes a great accompaniment to these sweet grilled kabobs.

Dinner

<u>Nutrients per serving:</u> (2 kabobs)

Calories	191	Carbohydrate	17 g
Calories from Fat	23 %	Cholesterol	53 mg
Total Fat	5 g	Sodium	183 mg
Saturated Fat	2 g	Dietary Fiber	1 g
Protein	19 g		

Dietary Exchanges: 1 Fruit, 2½ Lean Meat, 1 Fat

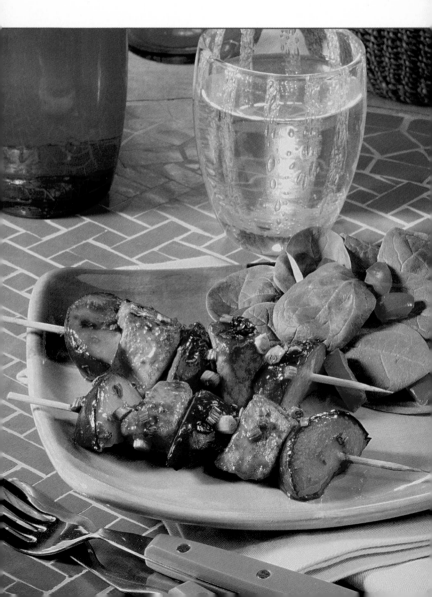

Teriyaki Salmon with Asian Slaw

Carb Friendly

4 tablespoons reduced-sodium teriyaki sauce, divided
2 boneless salmon fillets with skin (about 4 to 5 ounces each and 1 inch thick)
2½ cups coleslaw mix
1 cup snow peas, cut into thin strips
½ cup thinly sliced radishes
2 tablespoons orange marmalade
1 teaspoon dark sesame oil

1. Preheat broiler or prepare grill for direct cooking. Spoon 2 tablespoons teriyaki sauce over fleshy sides of salmon. Let stand while preparing vegetable mixture.

2. Combine coleslaw mix, snow peas and radishes in large bowl. Combine remaining 2 tablespoons teriyaki sauce, marmalade and sesame oil in small bowl. Add to coleslaw mixture; toss well.

3. Broil salmon 4 to 5 inches from heat, or grill flesh side down over medium coals 6 to 10 minutes or until center is opaque and fish just begins to flake when tested with fork. Transfer coleslaw mixture to serving plates; serve with salmon. *Makes 2 servings*

Nutrients per serving: (1 salmon fillet with 2 cups slaw)

Calories	327	Carbohydrate	22 g
Calories from Fat	41%	Cholesterol	67 mg
Total Fat	15 g	Sodium	615 mg
Saturated Fat	3 g	Dietary Fiber	3 g
Protein	25 g		

Dietary Exchanges: ½ Starch, 3 Vegetable, 4 Lean Meat, 3 Fat

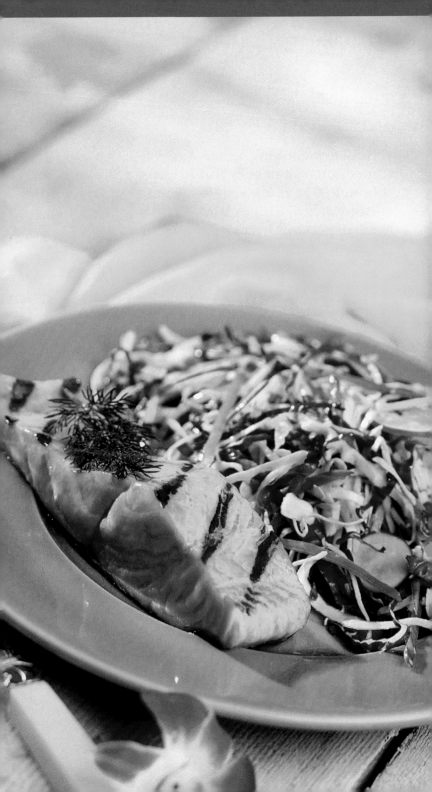

Sirloin with Sweet Caramelized Onions

Nonstick cooking spray
1 medium onion, very thinly sliced
1 boneless beef top sirloin steak (about 1 pound)
¼ cup water
2 tablespoons Worcestershire sauce
1 tablespoon sugar

1. Lightly coat 12-inch skillet with cooking spray; heat over high heat. Add onion; cook and stir 4 minutes or until browned. Remove from skillet and set aside. Wipe out skillet with paper towel.

2. Coat same skillet with cooking spray; heat over medium-high heat. Add beef; cook 10 to 13 minutes for medium-rare to medium, turning once. Remove from heat and transfer steak to cutting board; let stand 3 minutes before slicing.

3. Meanwhile, return skillet to high heat; add onion, water, Worcestershire sauce and sugar. Cook 30 to 45 seconds or until most liquid has evaporated.

4. Thinly slice beef on the diagonal; serve with onions.

Makes 4 servings

Nutrients per serving: (¼ of total recipe)

Calories	159	Carbohydrate	7 g
Calories from Fat	28%	Cholesterol	60 mg
Total Fat	5 g	Sodium	118 mg
Saturated Fat	2 g	Dietary Fiber	1 g
Protein	21 g		

Dietary Exchanges: ½ Starch, 3 Lean Meat, 1 Fat

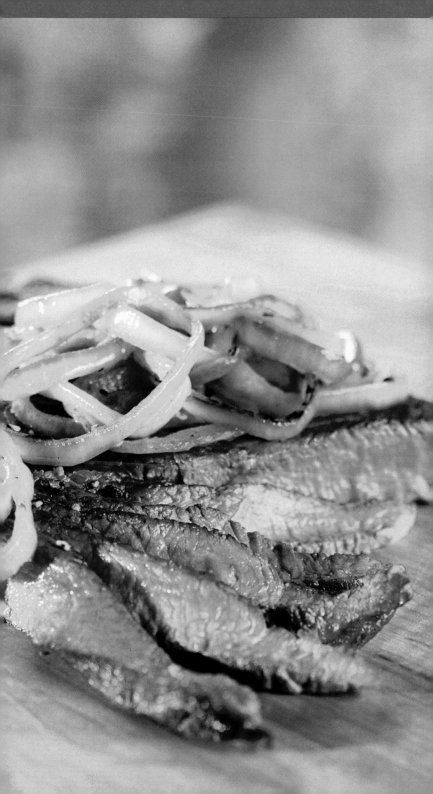

Lime-Mustard
Marinated Chicken

  **2 boneless skinless chicken breasts (about
     $\frac{1}{4}$ pound each)**
$\frac{1}{4}$ **cup fresh lime juice**
  3 tablespoons honey mustard, divided
  2 teaspoons olive oil
$\frac{1}{4}$ **teaspoon ground cumin**
$\frac{1}{8}$ **teaspoon garlic powder**
$\frac{1}{8}$ **teaspoon ground red pepper**
$\frac{3}{4}$ **cup plus 2 tablespoons fat-free reduced-
     sodium chicken broth, divided**
$\frac{1}{4}$ **cup uncooked rice**
  1 cup broccoli florets
$\frac{1}{3}$ **cup matchstick-size carrots**

1. Place chicken in large resealable food storage bag.
Whisk together lime juice, 2 tablespoons mustard, oil,
cumin, garlic powder and red pepper. Pour mixture
over chicken in bag. Seal bag; turn to coat. Marinate in
refrigerator 2 hours.

2. Combine ¾ cup broth, rice and remaining 1 tablespoon
mustard in small saucepan. Bring to a boil over high
heat. Reduce heat. Cover; simmer 12 minutes or until rice
is almost tender. Stir in broccoli, carrots and remaining
2 tablespoons broth. Cook, covered, 2 to 3 minutes more
or until vegetables are crisp-tender and rice is tender.

3. Meanwhile, prepare grill for direct cooking. Drain
chicken; discard marinade. Grill chicken over medium
heat, turning once, 10 to 13 minutes or until cooked
through and no longer pink in center. Serve chicken with
rice mixture. *Makes 2 servings*

Dinner

Nutrients per serving: (1 breast)

Calories	250	Carbohydrate	25 g
Calories from Fat	8 %	Cholesterol	66 mg
Total Fat	2 g	Sodium	393 mg
Saturated Fat	<1 g	Dietary Fiber	2 g
Protein	31 g		

Dietary Exchanges: 1 Starch, 2 Vegetable, 4 Lean Meat

Shrimp and Pineapple Kabobs

½ **pound medium raw shrimp, peeled and**
  deveined
½ **cup pineapple juice**
¼ **teaspoon garlic powder**
12 **chunks canned pineapple (in own juice)**
 1 **green bell pepper, cut into 1-inch pieces**
¼ **cup prepared chili sauce**

1. Combine shrimp, ½ cup pineapple juice and garlic powder in medium bowl; toss to coat. Marinate in refrigerator 30 minutes. Drain shrimp; discard marinade.

2. Alternately thread pineapple, pepper and shrimp onto 4 (10-inch) skewers. Brush with chili sauce. Grill 4 inches from heat 5 minutes or until shrimp are opaque, turning once and basting with chili sauce.   *Makes 4 servings*

Nutrients per serving: (1 kabob)

Calories	100	Carbohydrate	14 g
Calories from Fat	7 %	Cholesterol	87 mg
Total Fat	<1 g	Sodium	302 mg
Saturated Fat	<1 g	Dietary Fiber	1 g
Protein	10 g		

Dietary Exchanges: ½ Fruit, 1 Vegetable, 1 Lean Meat

Sides

∽

Green Beans and Red Onion with Mustard Vinaigrette Dressing ⭐ Carb Friendly

1½ pounds fresh green beans, trimmed
1 cup sliced red onion
3 tablespoons red wine vinegar
2 tablespoons Dijon mustard
1 tablespoon olive oil
¼ teaspoon salt
¼ teaspoon black pepper

1. Cook green beans in boiling water 8 minutes or until crisp-tender. Drain. Combine green beans and onion in large bowl.

2. Whisk together vinegar, mustard, oil, salt and pepper in microwavable bowl. Microwave on HIGH 1 minute. Whisk again.

3. Drizzle dressing over bean mixture. Toss well to coat.

Makes 6 servings

Nutrients per serving: (1 cup)

Calories	68	Carbohydrate	10 g
Calories from Fat	31%	Cholesterol	0 mg
Total Fat	2 g	Sodium	219 mg
Saturated Fat	<1 g	Dietary Fiber	4 g
Protein	2 g		

Dietary Exchanges: 2 Vegetable, ½ Fat

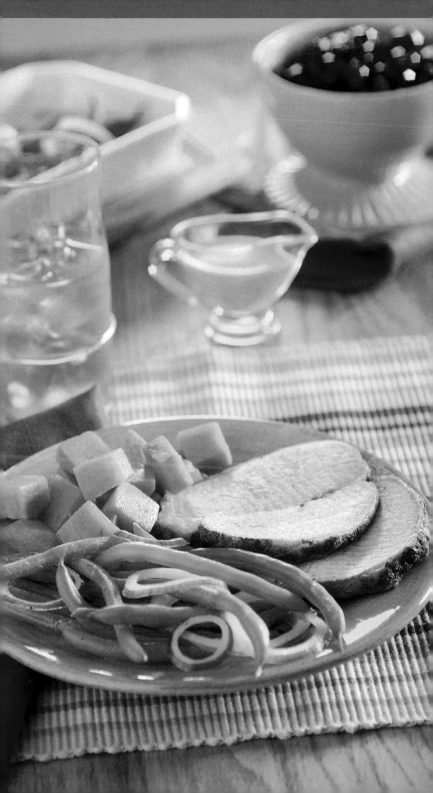

Light Lemon Cauliflower

Carb Friendly

4 tablespoons chopped fresh parsley, divided
½ teaspoon grated lemon peel
6 cups (about 1½ pounds) cauliflower florets
1 tablespoon reduced-fat margarine
3 cloves garlic, minced
2 tablespoons lemon juice
¼ cup grated Parmesan cheese
   Lemon slices (optional)

1. Place 1 tablespoon parsley, lemon peel and about 1 inch water in large saucepan. Place cauliflower in steamer basket; place in saucepan. Bring water to a boil over medium heat. Cover; steam 14 to 16 minutes or until cauliflower is crisp-tender. Remove to large bowl; keep warm. Reserve ½ cup hot liquid.

2. For sauce, heat margarine in small saucepan over medium heat. Add garlic; cook and stir 2 to 3 minutes or until soft. Stir in lemon juice and reserved liquid.

3. Spoon sauce over cauliflower. Sprinkle with remaining 3 tablespoons parsley and cheese before serving. Garnish with lemon slices. *Makes 6 servings*

<u>**Nutrients per serving:**</u> (about ⅔ cup cauliflower with 1½ tablespoons sauce and 2 teaspoons cheese)

Calories	53	Carbohydrate	6 g
Calories from Fat	33 %	Cholesterol	3 mg
Total Fat	2 g	Sodium	116 mg
Saturated Fat	1 g	Dietary Fiber	3 g
Protein	4 g		

Dietary Exchanges: 1 Vegetable, ½ Lean Meat, ½ Fat

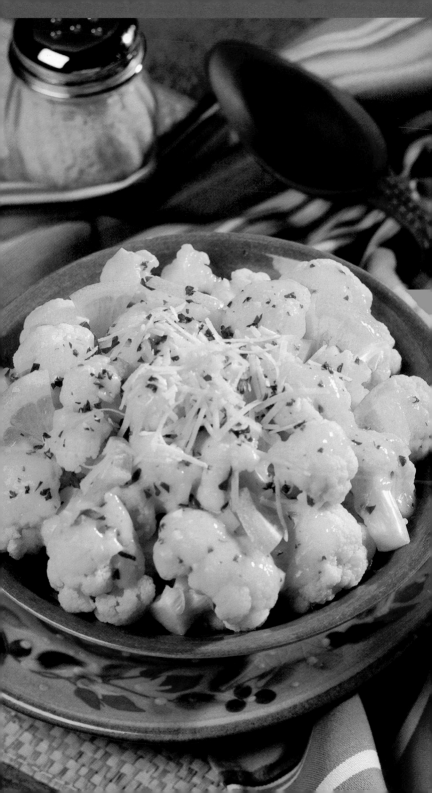

Sides

Potato-Cabbage Cakes

½ **cup refrigerated fat-free shredded hash brown potatoes**

½ **cup lightly packed coleslaw mix**

¼ **cup cholesterol-free egg substitute** *or* **2 egg whites**

¼ **teaspoon white pepper**

Nonstick cooking spray

4 **tablespoons unsweetened applesauce (optional)**

2 **tablespoons fat-free sour cream (optional)**

1. Mix hash browns, coleslaw mix, egg substitute and pepper in medium bowl. Pack half of hash brown mixture into ½-cup measure.

2. Spray large nonstick skillet with cooking spray; place over medium-high heat.

3. Gently invert cup into skillet. Repeat with remaining hash brown mixture. Drizzle any juices from bowl over cakes. When cakes begin to sizzle, gently press with spatula to flatten to ½-inch thickness and 4 inches in diameter. Cook 4 to 5 minutes per side or until cakes brown.

4. Top each cake with applesauce or sour cream, if desired. *Makes 2 servings*

Nutrients per serving: (1 cake)

Calories	82	**Carbohydrate**	17 g
Calories from Fat	0 %	**Cholesterol**	0 mg
Total Fat	0 g	**Sodium**	74 mg
Saturated Fat	0 g	**Dietary Fiber**	2 g
Protein	5 g		

Dietary Exchanges: 1 Starch, ½ Lean Meat

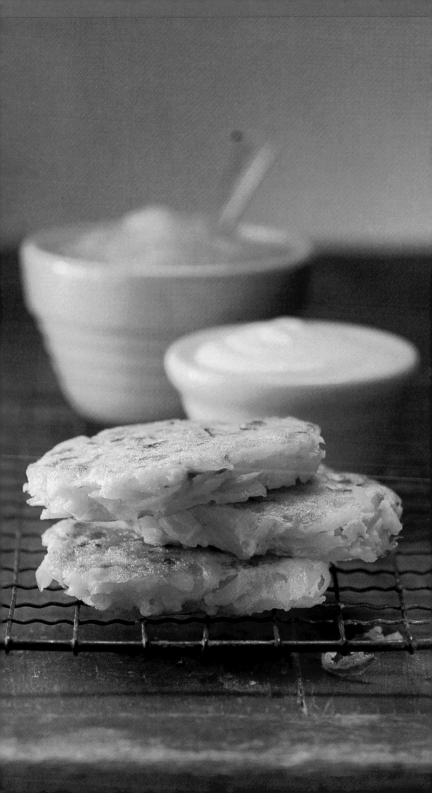

Pepper and Squash Gratin

1 russet potato (12 ounces), unpeeled
8 ounces yellow summer squash, thinly sliced
8 ounces zucchini, thinly sliced
2 cups frozen bell pepper stir-fry blend, thawed
1 teaspoon dried oregano
½ teaspoon salt
⅛ teaspoon black pepper (optional)
½ cup grated Parmesan cheese or shredded
    reduced-fat sharp Cheddar cheese
1 tablespoon butter or margarine, cut into
    8 pieces

1. Preheat oven to 375°F. Spray 12×8-inch glass baking dish with nonstick cooking spray. Pierce potato several times with fork. Microwave on HIGH 3 minutes. Cut potato into thin slices.

2. Layer half of potato, yellow squash, zucchini, bell pepper stir-fry blend, oregano, salt, black pepper, if desired, and cheese in prepared baking dish. Repeat layers. Dot with butter.

3. Cover tightly with foil; bake 25 minutes or until vegetables are just tender. Remove foil; bake 10 minutes more or until lightly browned. *Makes 8 servings*

Nutrients per serving: (⅛ of total recipe)

Calories	106	Carbohydrate	15 g
Calories from Fat	26%	Cholesterol	8 mg
Total Fat	3 g	Sodium	267 mg
Saturated Fat	2 g	Dietary Fiber	2 g
Protein	4 g		

Dietary Exchanges: 1 Starch, ½ Lean Meat, ½ Fat

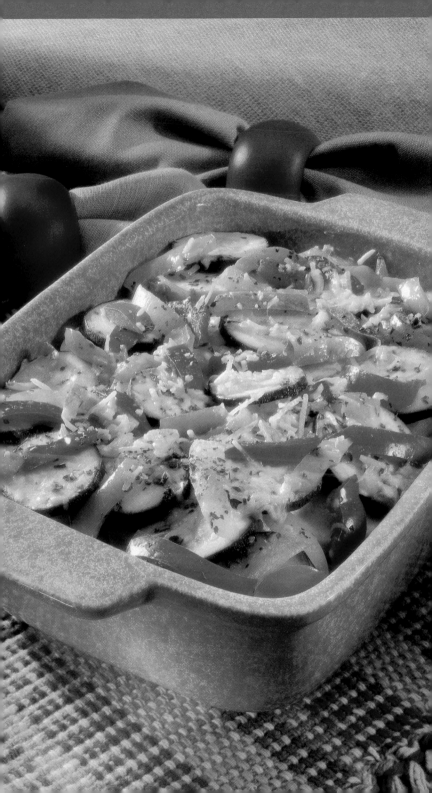

Tart & Tangy Cherry Salad

Carb Friendly

1 cup sugar-free lemon-lime soda
1 package (4-serving size) sugar-free cherry gelatin
1 can (14½ ounces) pitted tart red cherries in water
1 can (11 ounces) mandarin orange segments in light syrup
¼ cup sugar substitute
1 container (8 ounces) fat-free whipped topping
¼ cup finely chopped walnuts

1. Pour soda into large microwavable bowl. Microwave on HIGH 1 minute.

2. Whisk in gelatin until completely dissolved. Drain liquid from cherries and oranges into gelatin mixture. Stir until well blended.

3. Smash cherries with potato masher or fork in medium bowl. Sprinkle sugar substitute over cherries; mix well.

4. Stir cherry mixture, whipped topping and walnuts into gelatin until well blended. Gently fold in oranges. Pour mixture into glass bowl. Refrigerate 2 hours or until firm.

Makes 10 servings

Hint: This recipe is perfect to make the day before and refrigerate overnight.

<u>**Nutrients per serving:**</u> (½ cup salad)

Calories	96	**Carbohydrate**	17 g
Calories from Fat	20 %	**Cholesterol**	0 mg
Total Fat	2 g	**Sodium**	48 mg
Saturated Fat	<1 g	**Dietary Fiber**	1 g
Protein	1 g		

Dietary Exchanges: 1 Fruit, ½ Fat

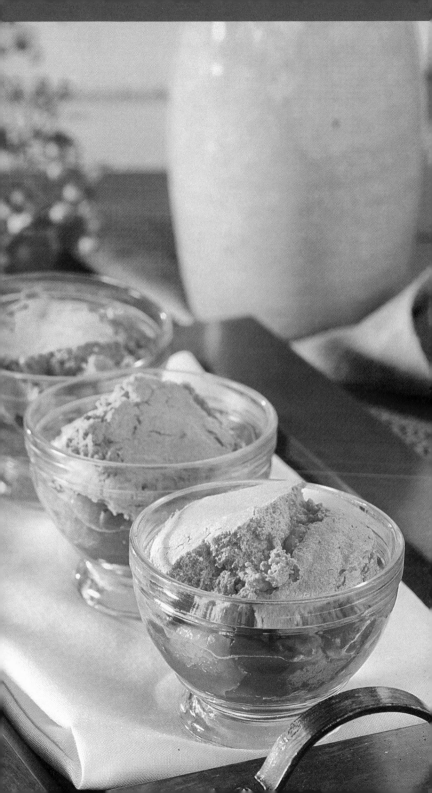

Sides

Creamy Lemon Gelatin with Blueberries

1 package (4-serving size) sugar-free lemon gelatin
½ cup boiling water
1 cup ice cubes
2 tablespoons lemon juice
1¼ cups vanilla fat-free yogurt
1 teaspoon grated lemon peel
½ cup frozen blueberries

1. Combine gelatin and boiling water in medium bowl; stir until gelatin is completely dissolved.

2. Add ice cubes and lemon juice; stir until ice cubes are melted and gelatin mixture is thickened. Remove and discard any unmelted ice.

3. Whisk in yogurt and lemon peel until completely smooth. Transfer mixture to 9-inch pie plate or decorative serving bowl. Cover with plastic wrap; refrigerate 1 hour or until firm.

4. Meanwhile, thaw blueberries in colander under cold running water. Drain on paper towels. Sprinkle blueberries over gelatin to serve.   *Makes 4 servings*

Nutrients per serving: (½ cup gelatin mixture with 2 tablespoons blueberries)

Calories	90	**Carbohydrate**	15 g
Calories from Fat	13 %	**Cholesterol**	5 mg
Total Fat	1 g	**Sodium**	108 mg
Saturated Fat	1 g	**Dietary Fiber**	1 g
Protein	4 g		

Dietary Exchanges: ½ Fruit, ½ Milk, ½ Lean Meat

Sides

Mashed Sweet Potatoes

2 large sweet potatoes (about 1¾ pounds)
¼ cup fat-free half-and-half
¾ teaspoon salt
¼ teaspoon ground cinnamon
⅛ teaspoon ground red pepper
¼ cup chopped pecans, toasted*

*To toast pecans, spread in shallow baking pan. Bake in preheated 350°F oven 5 to 7 minutes or until fragrant, stirring occasionally.

1. Peel potatoes; cut into chunks. Place in medium saucepan; cover with water. Cover; bring to a boil over high heat. Reduce heat to low; simmer about 15 minutes or until potatoes are tender. Drain; return to pan.

2. Add half-and-half, salt, cinnamon and red pepper. Mash with potato masher. Top with pecans.

Makes 6 servings

Nutrients per serving: (½ cup potatoes with 2 teaspoons pecans)

Calories	152	**Carbohydrate**	28 g
Calories from Fat	19 %	**Cholesterol**	2 mg
Total Fat	3 g	**Sodium**	370 mg
Saturated Fat	<1 g	**Dietary Fiber**	4 g
Protein	3 g		

Dietary Exchanges: 2 Starch, ½ Fat

Sides

Broccoli Supreme

2 packages (10 ounces each) frozen chopped broccoli
1 cup fat-free reduced-sodium chicken or vegetable broth
2 tablespoons reduced-fat mayonnaise
2 teaspoons dried minced onion (optional)

1. Combine broccoli, chicken broth, mayonnaise and onion, if desired, in large saucepan. Simmer, covered, stirring occasionally, until broccoli is tender.

2. Uncover; continue to simmer, stirring occasionally, until liquid has evaporated. *Makes 7 servings*

Nutrients per serving: (about ¾ cup broccoli)

Calories	31	**Carbohydrate**	4 g
Calories from Fat	25 %	**Cholesterol**	1 mg
Total Fat	1 g	**Sodium**	26 mg
Saturated Fat	<1 g	**Dietary Fiber**	2 g
Protein	2 g		

Dietary Exchanges: 1 Vegetable

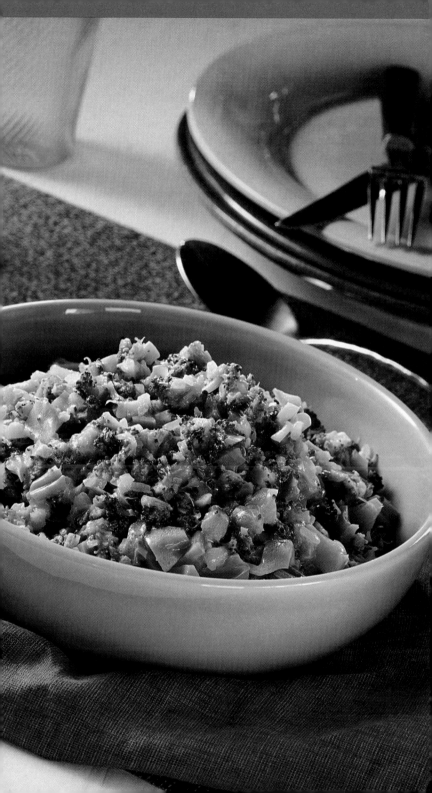

Sides

Brussels Sprouts with Walnuts

Carb Friendly

1 cup diced butternut squash (1-inch cubes)
1 pound brussels sprouts, trimmed
2 cups water
1 cup apple juice
½ cup fat-free vinaigrette salad dressing
1 cup arugula or baby spinach leaves
½ cup chopped walnuts, toasted*

*To toast walnuts, spread in shallow baking pan. Bake in preheated 350°F oven 5 to 7 minutes or until fragrant, stirring occasionally.

1. Preheat oven to 400°F. Lightly coat baking sheet with nonstick cooking spray. Roast squash on baking sheet 20 minutes or until tender; cool 5 minutes.

2. Meanwhile, combine brussels sprouts, water and apple juice in medium saucepan. Simmer over medium heat 15 minutes or until brussels sprouts are tender. Rinse under cold water; drain well. Cool 3 minutes.

3. Slice brussels sprouts lengthwise into thin slices. Mix with warm squash. Toss with salad dressing.

4. Divide greens among 4 plates. Spoon vegetables over greens. Sprinkle with walnuts.   *Makes 4 servings*

Nutrients per serving: (1 cup)

Calories	190	Carbohydrate	20 g
Calories from Fat	39 %	Cholesterol	0 mg
Total Fat	10 g	Sodium	204 mg
Saturated Fat	1 g	Dietary Fiber	6 g
Protein	7 g		

Dietary Exchanges: 1 Starch, ½ Fruit, 1 Lean Meat, 2 Fat

Garden Vegetable Scramble

2 medium ears corn
3 cups shredded green cabbage
2 medium zucchini, chopped
3 medium banana peppers, chopped *or* 1 large
    yellow or red bell pepper, chopped
1 large onion, chopped
1 tablespoon plus 2 teaspoons corn oil
2 tablespoons water
½ teaspoon salt
⅛ teaspoon red pepper flakes
3 large tomatoes, peeled and chopped
⅛ teaspoon black pepper

1. Cut corn kernels from cobs; place in large bowl. Add cabbage, zucchini, peppers and onion.

2. Heat oil in 12-inch skillet. Add vegetables; cook and stir 5 minutes. Add water, salt and red pepper flakes. Cover; simmer over low heat 15 to 20 minutes or until vegetables are tender. Stir in tomatoes and black pepper. Cook and stir 1 minute. *Makes 12 servings*

Nutrients per serving: (½ cup)

Calories	47	Carbohydrate	7 g
Calories from Fat	34 %	Cholesterol	0 mg
Total Fat	2 g	Sodium	107 mg
Saturated Fat	<1 g	Dietary Fiber	2 g
Protein	2 g		

Dietary Exchanges: ½ Starch, ½ Fat

Asparagus with No-Cook Creamy Mustard Sauce

½ cup plain fat-free yogurt
2 tablespoons reduced-fat mayonnaise
1 tablespoon Dijon mustard
2 teaspoons lemon juice
½ teaspoon salt
2 cups water
1½ pounds asparagus spears, trimmed
⅛ teaspoon black pepper (optional)

1. For sauce, whisk together yogurt, mayonnaise, mustard, lemon juice and salt in small bowl until smooth; set aside.

2. Bring water to a boil in 12-inch skillet over high heat. Add asparagus. Return to a boil. Reduce heat; cover and simmer 3 minutes or until crisp-tender. Drain on paper towels.

3. Place asparagus on serving platter; top with sauce. Sprinkle with pepper, if desired.   *Makes 6 servings*

<u>**Nutrients per serving:**</u> (about 6 asparagus spears with 2 tablespoons sauce)

Calories	57	Carbohydrate	8 g
Calories from Fat	28%	Cholesterol	2 mg
Total Fat	2 g	Sodium	299 mg
Saturated Fat	<1 g	Dietary Fiber	2 g
Protein	4 g		

Dietary Exchanges: 2 Vegetable, ½ Lean Meat

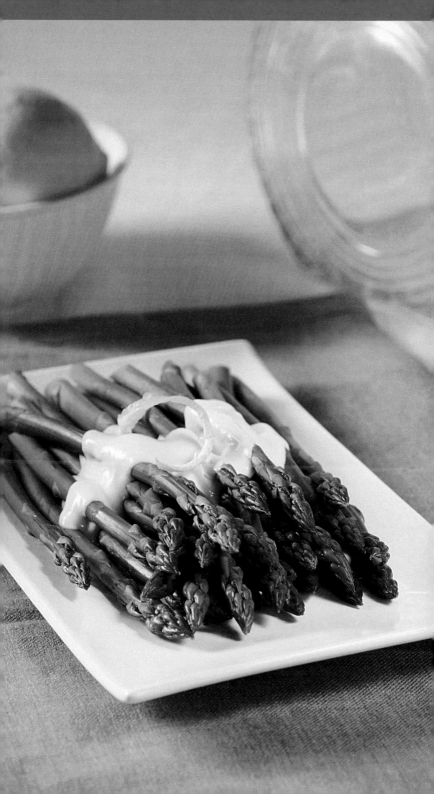

Dessert

No-Bake Cherry Cake

1 (10-inch) prepared angel food cake
1½ cups fat-free (skim) milk
1 cup reduced-fat sour cream
1 package (4-serving size) vanilla fat-free
    sugar-free instant pudding and pie filling
    mix
1 can (21 ounces) cherry pie filling

1. Tear cake into bite-size pieces; press into 11×7-inch baking dish.

2. Combine milk, sour cream and pudding mix in medium bowl; beat with wire whisk or electric mixer at medium speed 2 minutes or until thickened. Spread over cake in baking dish.

3. Spoon cherry pie filling evenly over top of cake. Chill; cut into 12 pieces to serve.   *Makes 12 servings*

Nutrients per serving: (1 piece [¹⁄₁₂ of cake])

Calories	156	Carbohydrate	31 g
Calories from Fat	11 %	Cholesterol	7 mg
Total Fat	2 g	Sodium	326 mg
Saturated Fat	1 g	Dietary Fiber	1 g
Protein	4 g		

Dietary Exchanges: 1 Starch, 1 Milk, ½ Lean Meat

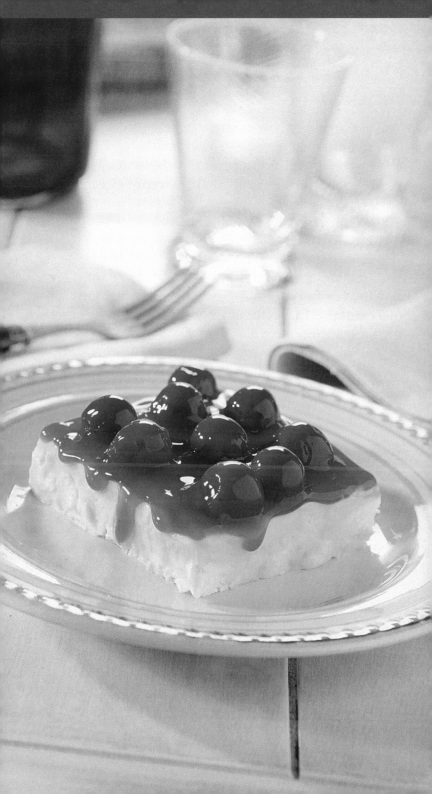

Grasshopper Pie

2 cups low-fat graham cracker crumbs
¼ cup unsweetened cocoa powder
¼ cup reduced-fat margarine, melted
1 package (8 ounces) fat-free cream cheese,
    softened
¼ cup sucralose-sugar blend
1 cup low-fat (1%) milk
1½ teaspoons vanilla
1 teaspoon mint extract
4 to 6 drops green food coloring (optional)
1 container (8 ounces) frozen fat-free whipped
    topping, thawed

1. Spray 9-inch pie plate with nonstick cooking spray. Combine cracker crumbs, cocoa and margarine in medium bowl. Press onto bottom and up side of prepared pie plate. Refrigerate.

2. Beat cream cheese and sucralose-sugar blend in large bowl with electric mixer at medium speed until fluffy. Gradually beat in milk until smooth. Stir in vanilla, mint extract and food coloring, if desired. Fold in whipped topping. Refrigerate 20 minutes or until chilled but not set. Pour into chilled crust. Freeze 4 hours or until set. Cut into 8 slices to serve. Freeze leftovers.

Makes 8 servings

Nutrients per serving: (1 slice [⅛ of pie])

Calories	271	Carbohydrate	33 g
Calories from Fat	27 %	Cholesterol	4 mg
Total Fat	8 g	Sodium	357 mg
Saturated Fat	2 g	Dietary Fiber	2 g
Protein	7 g		

Dietary Exchanges: 2 Starch, ½ Milk, 1 Lean Meat, 1½ Fat

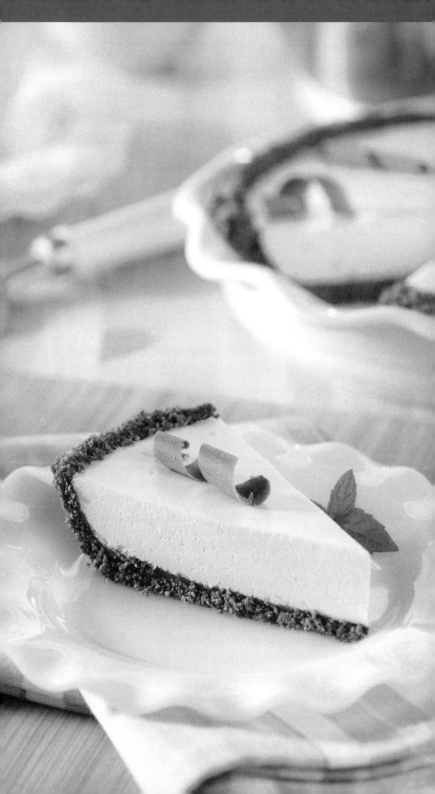

Chocolate-Orange Cake Roll

⅓ cup all-purpose flour, plus additional for
    dusting
¼ cup plus 1 tablespoon unsweetened cocoa
    powder, divided
¼ teaspoon baking soda
4 eggs, separated
½ teaspoon vanilla
¼ cup sugar substitute*
½ cup plus 2 tablespoons granulated sugar,
    divided
½ cup orange fruit spread

*This recipe was tested with sucralose-based sugar
substitute.*

1. Preheat oven to 375°F. Spray 15×10-inch jelly-roll pan
with nonstick cooking spray; dust with flour. Set aside.

2. Combine ⅓ cup flour, ¼ cup cocoa and baking soda in
small bowl; set aside.

3. Beat egg yolks and vanilla in large bowl with electric
mixer at high speed 5 minutes or until pale yellow. Beat
in sugar substitute and 2 tablespoons granulated sugar.

4. Beat egg whites in another large bowl at high speed
until soft peaks form. Beat in remaining ½ cup granulated
sugar until stiff peaks form.

5. Fold egg yolk mixture into egg white mixture. Sift flour
mixture over top; fold flour mixture into egg mixture
just until blended. Spread in prepared pan. Bake 12 to
15 minutes or until top springs back when lightly touched.

6. Meanwhile, sprinkle remaining 1 tablespoon cocoa
onto clean kitchen towel. Loosen cake from pan; invert

Dessert

onto prepared towel. Roll up towel and cake, starting from a short side. Cool on wire rack.

7. Unroll cake; remove towel. Top with orange fruit spread. Roll up cake. Cut into 10 slices to serve.

Makes 10 servings

Nutrients per serving: (1 slice [¹⁄₁₀ of cake roll])

Calories	136	Carbohydrate	25 g
Calories from Fat	15 %	Cholesterol	85 mg
Total Fat	2 g	Sodium	60 mg
Saturated Fat	1 g	Dietary Fiber	1 g
Protein	3 g		

Dietary Exchanges: 1½ Starch, ½ Fruit, ½ Fat

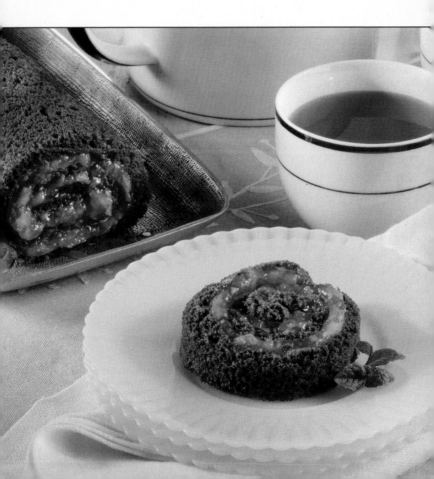

Dessert

Pumpkin Tartlets

½ (15-ounce) package refrigerated pie crusts
1 can (15 ounces) solid-pack pumpkin (not pumpkin pie filling)
¼ cup fat-free (skim) milk
1 egg
3 tablespoons sugar substitute*
3 tablespoons granulated sugar
¾ teaspoon ground cinnamon
½ teaspoon vanilla
⅛ teaspoon salt
⅛ teaspoon ground nutmeg
Dash ground allspice
1½ cups fat-free whipped topping

This recipe was tested with sucralose-based sugar substitute.

1. Preheat oven to 425°F. Spray 12 standard (2½-inch) muffin cups with nonstick cooking spray; set aside.

2. Unroll pie crust on clean work surface. Cut 12 circles with 2½-inch biscuit cutter; discard scraps. Press 1 circle into each prepared muffin cup.

3. Combine pumpkin, milk, egg, sugar substitute, granulated sugar, cinnamon, vanilla, salt, nutmeg and allspice in medium bowl; mix well. Spoon about 2 tablespoons pumpkin mixture into each tartlet shell. Bake 10 minutes.

4. *Reduce heat to 325°F.* Bake 12 to 15 minutes more or until knife inserted into tartlet centers comes out clean. Remove to wire rack; cool completely. Dollop 2 tablespoons whipped topping onto each tartlet just before serving. *Makes 12 servings*

Dessert

Nutrients per serving: (1 tartlet)

Calories	205	Carbohydrate	27 g
Calories from Fat	43 %	Cholesterol	24 mg
Total Fat	10 g	Sodium	183 mg
Saturated Fat	4 g	Dietary Fiber	1 g
Protein	2 g		

Dietary Exchanges: 2 Starch, 2 Fat

Peaches & Cream Freeze

1 package (8 ounces) reduced-fat cream cheese
1 cup fat-free sour cream
2½ teaspoons sugar substitute
2 teaspoons lemon juice
7 cups coarsely chopped peeled peaches
12 pecan halves (optional)

1. Line 12 standard (2½-inch) muffin cups with paper baking cups. Beat cream cheese, sour cream, sugar substitute and lemon juice in medium bowl with electric mixer at medium speed until smooth. Stir in peaches.

2. Spoon ½ cup mixture into each prepared muffin cup. Garnish with pecan halves, if desired. Cover; freeze 6 hours or until firm. Let stand at room temperature 10 minutes or until slightly softened before serving.

Makes 12 servings

Nutrients per serving: (½ cup freeze)

Calories	116	Carbohydrate	24 g
Calories from Fat	5 %	Cholesterol	5 mg
Total Fat	1 g	Sodium	120 mg
Saturated Fat	0 g	Dietary Fiber	3 g
Protein	6 g		

Dietary Exchanges: 1 Starch, 1 Fruit, 1 Lean Meat

Light Latte Cookies

1¾ cups all-purpose flour
¼ cup unsweetened cocoa powder
1 tablespoon plus 1 teaspoon instant
    decaffeinated coffee granules, divided
1 teaspoon baking soda
½ teaspoon ground cinnamon
½ cup (1 stick) soft baking butter with canola oil
½ cup packed dark brown sugar
¼ cup fat-free sour cream
1 egg
1 egg white
1 teaspoon vanilla
¾ cup powdered sugar
1 to 2 tablespoons fat-free (skim) milk
Additional powdered sugar (optional)

1. Preheat oven to 350°F. Combine flour, cocoa, 1 tablespoon coffee granules, baking soda and cinnamon in large bowl; set aside.

2. Beat butter in another large bowl with electric mixer at medium speed 30 seconds or until creamy. Beat in brown sugar and sour cream until well blended. Add egg, egg white and vanilla; beat at low speed until well blended. Gradually add flour mixture, beating at low speed until well blended.

3. Drop dough by level teaspoonfuls onto ungreased cookie sheets. Flatten slightly with bottom of greased glass. Bake 6 minutes. Cool 5 minutes on cookie sheets. Remove to wire racks; cool completely.

4. For icing, stir together ¾ cup powdered sugar and enough milk to reach drizzling consistency. Drizzle over

Dessert

cookies. Let stand until icing is firm. Dust with additional powdered sugar, if desired. *Makes 6 dozen cookies*

Nutrients per serving: (2 cookies)

Calories	74	**Carbohydrate**	11 g
Calories from Fat	34 %	**Cholesterol**	11 mg
Total Fat	3 g	**Sodium**	62 mg
Saturated Fat	1 g	**Dietary Fiber**	<1 g
Protein	1 g		

Dietary Exchanges: 1 Starch

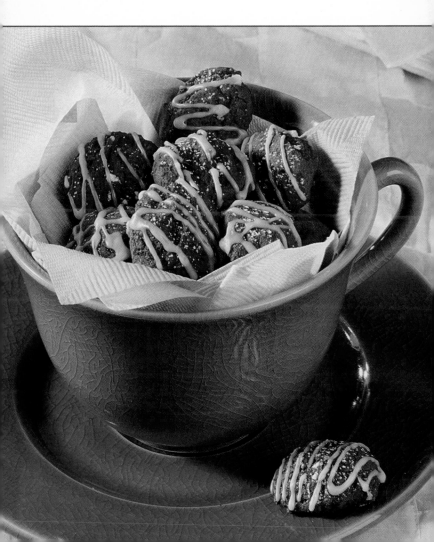

Lemon Cream Peach and Blueberry Pie

2 cups low-fat (1%) milk
¼ cup cholesterol-free egg substitute
3 tablespoons cornstarch
⅛ teaspoon salt
7 packets sucralose-based sugar substitute
3 tablespoons lemon juice
1 teaspoon grated lemon peel
1 teaspoon vanilla
1 (6-ounce) prepared graham cracker crust
1 cup fresh or thawed frozen peach slices
¾ cup fresh or frozen blueberries, thawed, rinsed and drained

1. Combine milk, egg substitute, cornstarch and salt in medium saucepan; whisk until cornstarch is dissolved. Cook over medium heat, stirring constantly, about 5 minutes or until mixture boils and thickens. Stir in sugar substitute, lemon juice, lemon peel and vanilla. Transfer mixture to medium bowl.

2. Place sheet of plastic wrap on top of filling to prevent skin from forming. Let mixture cool to room temperature. Spoon into crust. Decoratively top with peaches and blueberries. Chill completely; slice into 8 wedges to serve. *Makes 8 servings*

Hint: Substitute any of your favorite in-season fruits for the peaches and blueberries.

Tip: Try cubing the peaches as a variation on the slices to create smaller bites for easier eating.

Dessert

Nutrients per serving: (1 wedge [⅛ of pie])

Calories	168	Carbohydrate	25 g
Calories from Fat	32 %	Cholesterol	3 mg
Total Fat	6 g	Sodium	200 mg
Saturated Fat	2 g	Dietary Fiber	1 g
Protein	4 g		

Dietary Exchanges: 1 Starch, ½ Fruit, ½ Milk, ½ Lean Meat, 1 Fat

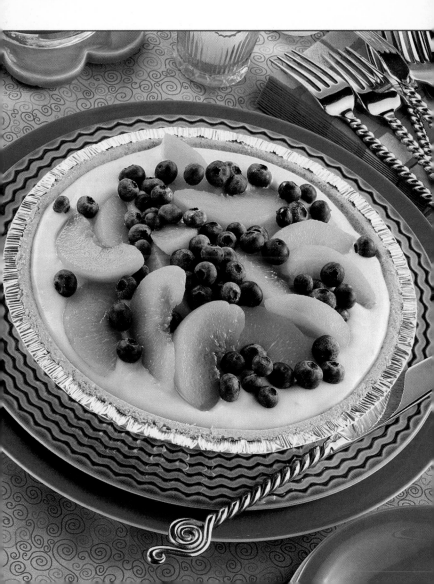

Streusel-Topped Strawberry Cheesecake Squares

1 container (8 ounces) strawberry sugar-free
    fat-free yogurt
1 package (8 ounces) fat-free cream cheese
½ (8-ounce) package reduced-fat cream cheese
¼ cup sucralose-based sugar substitute
1 envelope (¼ ounce) unflavored gelatin
2 tablespoons water
1 cup chopped fresh strawberries
1 tablespoon granulated sugar
1 cup sliced fresh strawberries
⅓ cup low-fat granola

1. Line 9-inch square baking pan with plastic wrap, leaving 4-inch overhang on 2 opposite sides.

2. Combine yogurt, cream cheese and sugar substitute in medium bowl; beat until smooth. Set aside.

3. Combine gelatin and water in small microwavable bowl; let stand 2 minutes. Microwave on HIGH 40 seconds to dissolve gelatin. Beat gelatin into yogurt mixture. Combine chopped strawberries and granulated sugar in small bowl. Add to yogurt mixture.

4. Pour yogurt mixture into prepared pan. Refrigerate 1 hour or until firm.

5. Arrange sliced strawberries over top just before serving; sprinkle evenly with granola.

6. Gently lift cheesecake out of pan with plastic wrap. Pull plastic wrap away from sides. Cut into 9 squares to serve. *Makes 9 servings*

Dessert

Nutrients per serving: (1 square [⅑ of cheesecake])

Calories	98	Carbohydrate	11 g
Calories from Fat	24 %	Cholesterol	8 mg
Total Fat	3 g	Sodium	223 mg
Saturated Fat	2 g	Dietary Fiber	1 g
Protein	7 g		

Dietary Exchanges: 1 Starch, ½ Fruit, ½ Milk, 1 Lean Meat, ½ Fat

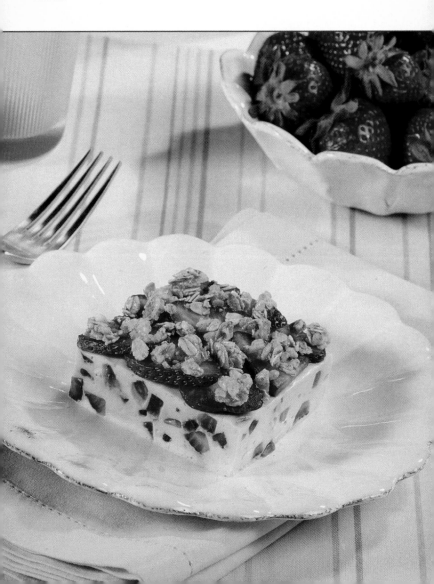

Dessert

Shortcake Cobbler

2 cups pear slices
**2 cups frozen unsweetened peach slices,
    partially thawed**
2 tablespoons raisins
¼ cup water
2 tablespoons sucralose-based sugar substitute
2 teaspoons cornstarch
**¼ teaspoon vanilla or vanilla, butter and nut
    flavoring**
1 cup reduced-fat biscuit baking mix
½ cup plain fat-free yogurt
2 tablespoons granulated sugar
2 tablespoons reduced-fat margarine, melted
1 teaspoon grated orange peel
¼ teaspoon ground cinnamon

1. Preheat oven to 425°F.

2. Spray 11×7-inch baking dish with nonstick cooking spray. Add pears, peaches and raisins; set aside.

3. Combine water, sugar substitute, cornstarch and vanilla in small bowl; stir until cornstarch dissolves. Pour over fruit mixture in baking dish; toss gently to coat.

4. Combine biscuit baking mix, yogurt, granulated sugar, margarine, orange peel and cinnamon in medium bowl; stir until well blended and mixture forms stiff batter. Spoon batter onto fruit mixture in 8 mounds. Bake 20 minutes or until topping is light brown. Serve warm or at room temperature. *Makes 8 servings*

Dessert

Nutrients per serving: (½ cup cobbler)

Calories	153	Carbohydrate	32 g
Calories from Fat	15 %	Cholesterol	<1 mg
Total Fat	3 g	Sodium	235 mg
Saturated Fat	<1 g	Dietary Fiber	3 g
Protein	3 g		

Dietary Exchanges: 1 Starch, 1 Fruit, ½ Fat

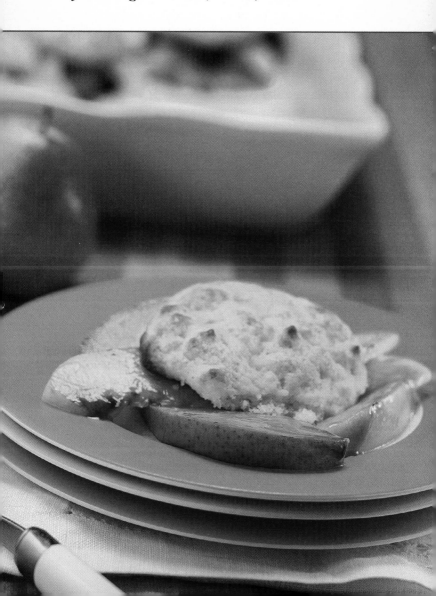

Dessert

Individual Pear Upside-Down Cakes

2 tablespoons no-sugar-added strawberry fruit spread

1 pear, halved, cored and very thinly sliced

¼ cup cake flour

1 tablespoon plus 1½ teaspoons sucralose-based sugar substitute, divided

3 egg whites

¼ teaspoon cream of tartar

½ teaspoon vanilla

MICROWAVE DIRECTIONS

1. Lightly spray 2 large (12-ounce) microwavable coffee cups with nonstick cooking spray. Place 1 tablespoon strawberry fruit spread in each cup. Layer pear slices over fruit spread. Set aside.

2. Sift together flour and 1 tablespoon sugar substitute in medium bowl; set aside.

3. Beat egg whites in large bowl with electric mixer at high speed until foamy. Add cream of tartar; beat until almost stiff. Gradually add remaining 1½ teaspoons sugar substitute. Beat at high speed 1 minute. Fold in vanilla, then flour mixture. Pour batter into prepared coffee cups. Microwave on HIGH 3 minutes. Turn cakes out onto dessert plates. Serve hot or cold.   *Makes 2 servings*

Nutrients per serving: (1 cake)

Calories	138	Carbohydrate	30 g
Calories from Fat	2 %	Cholesterol	0 mg
Total Fat	<1 g	Sodium	85 mg
Saturated Fat	<1 g	Dietary Fiber	3 g
Protein	7 g		

Dietary Exchanges: 1 Starch, 1 Fruit, 1 Lean Meat

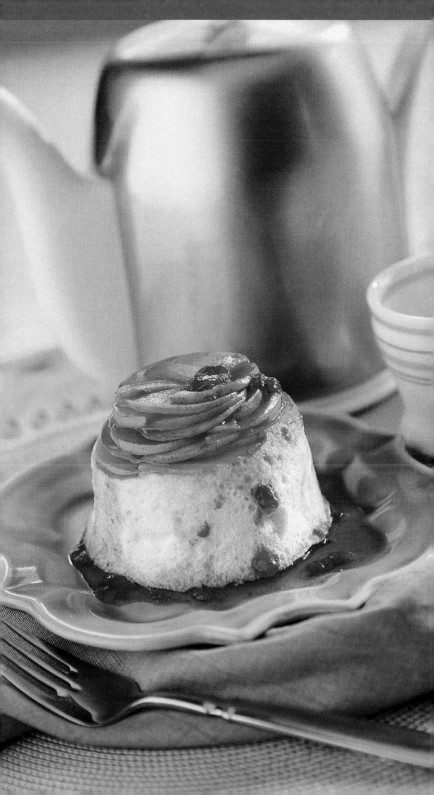

Chocolate-Strawberry Layer Cake

1½ cups all-purpose flour
¾ cup sucralose-sugar blend
1 teaspoon baking powder
1 teaspoon baking soda
¼ teaspoon salt
1 cup water
⅓ cup unsweetened cocoa powder
2 tablespoons butter
½ teaspoon instant espresso powder or instant coffee powder (optional)
⅓ cup low-fat buttermilk
⅓ cup cholesterol-free egg substitute
3 tablespoons canola oil
2 teaspoons vanilla
⅓ cup sugar-free strawberry preserves
¾ cup frozen fat-free whipped topping, thawed
Additional fat-free whipped topping, thawed (optional)
Fresh strawberry slices (optional)
¼ square (¼ ounce) semisweet chocolate, grated (optional)

1. Preheat oven to 350°F. Coat 2 (8-inch) round baking pans with nonstick cooking spray. Line bottoms of pans with parchment paper or waxed paper; set aside.

2. Combine flour, sucralose-sugar blend, baking powder, baking soda and salt in large bowl. Combine water, cocoa powder, butter and espresso, if desired, in small saucepan. Cook, stirring constantly, over medium heat until butter melts. Remove from heat; let stand 5 minutes.

3. Gradually add water mixture to dry ingredients with electric mixer at low speed, beating just until combined. (Do not overmix.) Add buttermilk, egg substitute, oil and vanilla; beat 1 minute at medium speed or until smooth. Pour into prepared pans.

4. Bake about 20 minutes or until toothpick inserted into centers comes out clean. Cool in pans on wire racks 5 minutes. Remove from pans; cool completely.

5. Place 1 cake layer, bottom side up, on cake plate. Stir strawberry preserves; spread over cake layer. Top with ¾ cup whipped topping. Place remaining cake layer, bottom side down, on top. Garnish with additional whipped topping, fresh strawberry slices and grated chocolate, if desired. Store leftovers in refrigerator.

Makes 16 servings

Nutrients per serving: (1 slice [$\frac{1}{16}$ of cake])

Calories	168	Carbohydrate	27 g
Calories from Fat	27 %	Cholesterol	4 mg
Total Fat	4 g	Sodium	181 mg
Saturated Fat	1 g	Dietary Fiber	1 g
Protein	1 g		

Dietary Exchanges: 1 Starch, 1 Milk, 1 Fat

Index

Index

Index